the woman with a worm in her head

and Other True Stories of Infectious Diseases

Pamela Nagami, M.D.

foreword by F. Gonzalez-Crussi

St. Martin's Griffin ᛘ New York

To Glenn

www.stmartins.com

Library of Congress Control Number: 2001095048
ISBN 0-312-30601-6

First published by Renaissance Books under the title *Maneater*

10 9 8 7 6 5 4 3

acknowledgments

I am grateful to my friends and family who read the manuscript and contributed suggestions and criticism: Wendy Herbert, Edward Power, Dr. Claire Panosian, and to Michelle Raffin for help with early rewrites. Thanks to my son, Paul Nagami, for help with the index and the glossary. For their expert clinical advice: Sue Partridge and Dr. Holly Williams at the Centers for Disease Control and Prevention, and Dr. Michel Philippart at the University of California at Los Angeles. For library support: Elliott M. Gordon, Marsha L. Edenburn, and Annette Wolfson. To the hospital and regional laboratories and, especially, to Edward Schackman, Ed Nugent, and Michael Collier. To the doctors, nurses, pharmacists, and all the trained professionals at my hospital, thank you.

Special thanks to my collaborator and teacher, Donna Frazier, to my indefatigable agent, B. J. Robbins, and to my editor, Richard O'Connor.

And to the patients and families of *The Woman with a Worm in Her Head.*

With the exception of the late Dr. Rasoul Soudmand, the patients, nurses, and doctors in my hospital who appear in *The Woman with a Worm in Her Head* have been given pseudonyms. Outside consultants appear under their own names.

contents

foreword

That many physicians feel compelled to express themselves through literary writing is generally known. Nor should this be a cause for wonderment or surprise. Physicians are placed on the front line, so to speak, of the mighty clash between forces that sustain human life and those that oppose it. By its very nature, their job forces them daily to canvass the conflict at the closest possible range. What they see is far from trivial: on the one hand, the will to live—the dumb striving, the unyielding impetus to survive; on the other, the frost that withers life, the ills that wear it down, the tempests that scathe it. And the physician stands in the midst of it all, a privileged spectator of every phase of this conflict. It is natural that he or she would feel the urge to describe, to record what is occurring. What for? To bear witness; to inform us; to spread hope and to console others, since this is, after all, a physician's calling. Sometimes to convey his/her genuine admiration for the unsurpassed magnificence of the observed phenomena. For the virtuosity of Nature may reveal itself unexpectedly in disease and appear no less admirable when perturbed than when sound. But the physician also writes as catharsis, to alleviate his own anguish. For all we know, this may be his main motive: a means to hold in suspense the misery that comes from glancing too intently on the chaos of the world.

The narratives developed in the present work reflect the experience of a physician who happens to be a specialist in infectious diseases. Her vantage point casts a light on all perceptions. But it is apparent that she is a physician first, and this in the most fundamental acceptation of the term: her professional life is spent in combat in the front line of the mighty struggle. The foe that she faces is overwhelmingly powerful. Bacteria, viruses, and fungi have a history of resiliency and survival that ought to humble the omnipresent pride of our species, if we so much as fleetingly consider the facts. Bacteria were present billions of years before there was any intimation of a human race, and it is a safe wager that they will be around long after the last trace of mankind has vanished.

Nothing in our technology can match this infrangible sturdiness, this amazing invulnerability, tested over eons of evolution. Against this foe, our efforts are powerless and our clever devices nugatory. We are forced to own that, in the long run, we shall lose the battle. But the physician, who is all except "defeatist," is unfazed by this, and does not adopt such a sweeping, philosophical viewpoint. He, or she, is not concerned with the destiny of the human race as a nameless, faceless, all-embracing totality. Or with what will happen in a future that is measured in the geological time scale. His concern is with human beings, here and now. Patients have names, and fears, and joys, and aspirations, and all these form part of the disease. Moreover, diseases never develop in a vacuum; least of all infectious diseases, whose contagiousness best epitomizes the social structure of human suffering. But transmissibility is only one among many factors through which suffering manages to reveal our ties to the community. Doctor Nagami knows this well, and she tells us about her frustration in having to take into consideration such things as the availability of long-term disability benefits for patients who badly need them. Were the physician to consider only the harmful bacteria, fungi, and viruses, his most fundamental role would be subverted. Social and economic conditions have a lot to do with causing the disease and spreading it to the population. For the infectious disease specialist, who bears the responsibility for the detection and control of epidemics, these factors acquire particular relevance.

At a grandiose scale, in the fullness of time, the microbes shall win the battle. And we know they are going to win it, too, in the brief span of our individual lives. For the latter must ineluctably come to an end, and often the proximate cause is an infection that might have been trivial but that the ravages of old age or other circumstances render lethal. By whatever means, in the end we shall be microbial fodder; consumed, perhaps, inside the earth, which has long been the rightful property of the ubiquitous Microbe. Agricultural fields are said to host over a billion bacterial cells per gram of soil. These microbes run the risk of turning the medical specialist into a detached, unfeeling observer; that is, a skeptic, if not a cynic.

And yet, how rewarding it is to confirm that the spirit that breathes in Dr. Nagami's pages evince none of these claudicating attitudes. The vigor of hope is preserved, even in the face of the final incapacity. The depth of a humane vision is maintained to the end. The physician's own failings and shortcomings (for there is a limit to medical skills, despite the much-vaunted progress) are made into a route of escape from a ruinous sense of superiority. Death cannot be abolished, but the doctor's ministrations can now retard it more effectively than ever before. Suffering cannot be deleted, but the current means to lessen its pangs exceed any previous measure.

And this is why we all enjoy the physician's chronicle of the mighty struggle. It is a war that concerns us all, whose episodes are always fascinating. All the more so when told, as in these pages, directly, truthfully, and clearly, by a front-line veteran.

—F. Gonzalez-Crussi
Emeritus Professor of Pathology
Chicago, IL, August 2001

introduction

I know things about the human body because I've looked at what lucky people never see.

In a lot of ways, my world of sense memories is like yours. Both of us can close our eyes and remember the softness of a baby's skin, the sweet, sharp smell of an orange being peeled, the feeling of the breath that dries the back of the throat in the middle of a run, the way the heart begins to pound. But because I'm a doctor who specializes in infectious diseases—a bugs and drugs doc—I also know the particular geography of the body under siege.

I've seen the way tissue killed by gas-producing bacteria crackles under the finger like a ball of cellophane. I know the smell of a staph infection (mousy, musty, rancid), and how to see the gaps that tell me there's a parasite living in your brain: gaps in words you want to say, gaps in a movement of your hand, gaps in your gait. I can tell some diseases by touch. If there's a lesion on your skin, I'll close my eyes and pet it with the flat part of my right index fingertip, the finger that can tell me if what lies below is alive or dead, patient or invader. As I stand beside a surgeon who's unwrapping an infected foot, I know that the tissue is dead around the edges if it's dark and dry, and I get close and sniff the whole thing inch by inch like a dog for the telltale smell of hidden pus. "Cut here," I say, or "this part's fine."

To know the body this way, changed by some of the deadliest infections on the planet, means entering it with my brain and my senses. My work takes me into the midst of the agents that carry diseases, ancient and new, and my job is to disarm or kill them before they kill you, or me. Some are very small, like HIV, the chickenpox virus, or the encephalitis viruses, like West Nile. Or larger, like the bacteria staph or strep. Some are big enough to see with the naked eye, like the fuzzy fungus that, when inhaled, causes Valley Fever. And some would be hard to miss, if only you knew you were looking for them, like the pork tapeworms that riddle the brain with holes.

Keeping this kind of company is scary at first. People don't line up in medical school to get intimate with AIDS, parasitic worms, and flesh-eating bacteria. The natural human impulse is to pull away and protect ourselves, and to think we're safe because we're not in some jungle, waiting for the next Ebola outbreak. But the truth is, in the big-city HMO where I work, I often get paged twenty or thirty times a day to size up infectious diseases that come from what we eat, what we breathe, what we touch, and where we go. The rare and mysterious cases I see walk into my hospital every day.

I wear purple high-tops for speed, and up to four beepers to keep me wired to the departments that need me. I talk fast because there's no time not to. If a patient is critically ill, I dispense instant advice on how to start treatment. Often I work like a detective, sifting through the evidence other doctors give me: the patients' symptoms, their lab tests, where they went on vacation. I ask dozens of questions: When exactly did the pain start? Were there chills? Did they eat a rare delicacy in a foreign country? Is their parakeet sick? I examine them like a crime scene, looking for clues: a pattern of dots on the skin, a whooshing sound in the heart, an enlarged spleen, a pale spot on the back of the eye. I read lists of blood test results, look for shadows on x-ray film, and see what grows in culture dishes.

The doctors who ask for my help don't expect me to perform an operation, or even a procedure, but they do want me to think. If a heart valve is infected, I try to think like a cardiologist. If someone has a brain worm, I pretend I'm a neurologist and track the worm by studying its habits and preferences. Often, I know the diagnosis from the first sentence of the patient's history. And sometimes I can't figure it out even after years of study.

Some of the patients I see are so sick that there are days I feel as though death is making rounds with me. And there's always the nagging fear that I could bring something dangerous home and spread it to my husband or my children. In our house, my stethoscope wasn't a toy the kids were allowed to play with. We understood that the barrier between home and my work is flimsy. When I took my toddler to the clinic with fever, she didn't just get an ear check and some amoxicillin like everybody else's kid. She got her blood drawn to make sure she didn't have the same bug my patient had in the ICU.

Through the years I've tried to play all this down because every member of my family, except me, has some symptoms of obsessive compulsive disorder. It's the ultimate irony for me to have gone into infectious diseases in a family prone to fear of germs. So I try to be casual: I eat stuff that falls on the floor and I'm not compulsive about hand washing.

Of course, I can't hide everything from them. They notice that I won't hike in the hills on certain days in the fall when the Valley Fever winds are up. And one spring, when there was a little epidemic of spinal meningitis, my kids had to line up in the kitchen and get vaccinated for a disease most people hadn't even heard of. Like it or not, a bracing amount of fear comes with the job.

But just beyond the fear is the fascination of solving the mystery of a sudden illness that's tearing its way through a body. I can't save all my patients, but I have not forgotten a single name, or failed to add the telling details of their cases to the running list of facts I keep in my brain to help me see the next case more clearly, and diagnose it more quickly.

We live with the illusion that technology has put a safety zone between us and the diseases I see every day, but we're all vulnerable. And because we're afraid to look, we don't learn to see the signs that can save us and the people we love.

I'd like to show you how I learned to look and, finally, understand some of the most dangerous infections we know. It's a process that started with a childhood worm hunt and led me to hundreds of cases I'll never forget, infections that have changed my patients and me in ways none of us could have imagined.

As you join me in the ER, the OR, and the ICU, you'll learn to see the way I do, and feel the reality of the people who decipher the cryptic traces that infections leave in the body. And if I'm lucky, you might even decide to take a simple action that could save a life—get a chickenpox shot, take malaria pills before a trip, or get an infected family member to the hospital while there's still time for someone like me to help them.

worm hunt

"Do you have time to listen to a case? It's my husband. I am very worried about him." It was a young internist from Vietnam, Dr. Vy Tran.

I had been in my office doing paperwork on a quiet afternoon in early March 1999 when my phone rang. Now I leaned back in my swivel chair and said, "Absolutely. Go ahead."

"You know we went home to Vietnam for three weeks last month; we got back on February 19. About four days later, Hanh came home from work sick. He didn't eat very much dinner, and he went to bed early. I put my hand on his forehead and he felt hot. So I took his temperature and it was 103."

Dr. Tran went on to tell me that every morning Hanh felt better and went to work, but every night the sickness came. One night he had hives all over his feet; another he was doubled over with pain and pressure in his liver. And there was always fever. He asked Vy to turn up the heat; he crawled under the covers; he wanted extra blankets.

Dr. Tran gave her husband antibiotics without effect. She checked his white blood cell count, which was only slightly elevated.

Then she decided to consult her father in Maryland, who had been a doctor in Vietnam.

"You must run tests for malaria," he said.

So Dr. Tran brought Hanh back to the lab for a thick and thin blood smear for malaria and for another complete blood count.

"The malaria smear was negative, Pam, but the white blood count was twenty-six thousand, and over half the white cells were eosinophils!" she said.

I sat up straight in my chair. The white blood cells called eosinophils are the gaudy outriders of the blood stream. Their name means "fond of the red dye eosin." When a drop of blood is stained with that dye and viewed under the microscope, the eosinophils sparkle against the pale pink background of the red cells. Scarlet granules fill the entire eosinophil. The granules contain tissue-destroying enzymes and act like hand grenades. Eosinophils attack anything foreign that gets into the body, like pollen grains and cat dander. They move into the tissues, stick to the foreign substance, and explode their granules against it. If this happens in the airways, the patient gets red runny eyes and starts sneezing and wheezing. In the United States, it's the eosinophils that put the BMWs in the allergists' driveways.

But eosinophils did not evolve over millions of years just to make our noses run. They are ancient worm hunters, specialized to defend the body against parasites like roundworms and flukes. In the developed world, where sanitation is good, eosinophils are usually peacetime warriors. They rarely number more than three hundred per cubic millimeter of blood. But Hanh Le had more than thirteen thousand. It was the highest count I had ever seen.

The army of eosinophils pouring out of his bone marrow had to be after worms, I thought; nothing else would bring them out in such numbers. And that meant I had to hunt worms, too.

"Vy," I said, "Don't worry. We're going to figure this out and take care of Hanh. But I need to go over your trip step by step." And that's what I did, by talking with Vy and then with her husband, then sifting their stories for clues that might lead to worms: raw food that might incubate them, contact with water or people who might carry them. To track a worm, you have to find the place where the life cycle of the worm becomes part of the life cycle of the human host.

It was a familiar process for me because worms, and worm hunting, had been part of my own life cycle since my parents sent me to Camp Wing-a-Roo, on the shores of Lake Erie, when I was eight years old. There was a grassy compound with a natural creek that was small enough to jump over if you took a running start, and we explored it in maroon shorts and white tee shirts with the camp name scripted on the front. There were all the usual activities: archery, horseback riding, arts and crafts—and one or two things that were not in the brochure. Worm hunting was one of them.

The counselors had planned a fishing trip, and when they gathered the evening before to collect night crawlers, they asked me, alone among the campers, to join them. I don't really know why they singled me out. Perhaps it was because I was a gangly tomboy who brought them tadpoles and water boatmen from the creek. I asked a lot of questions. Whatever it was they saw, they got it right. I was thrilled by their invitation.

We gathered up flashlights, screwdrivers, and jars of mustard powder and water, and headed into the dark, feeling for the little heaped up mounds of dirt under the grass at the tops of the earthworm burrows. Then we pried off the turf with a screwdriver and poured mustard water into the holes.

Soon the worms began to emerge from their dens—long, glistening, and fat, the tiny bristles on their sides grabbing the earth one last time as we pulled them away and into a waiting can. Whether or not we caught any fish I don't remember, but after that I was hooked on worms—and though it seems odd, they've touched my life at key points. My first real kiss took place in the shrubbery of a botanical garden when a boy in junior high, knowing my weakness, lured me there under the pretext of finding flatworms in the stream. In high school, I dabbled in art—only instead of people or landscapes I sketched snails.

By the time I got to college I was headed for a life of field work and laboratory research. I spent countless hours at the seashore at low tide wading through the fetid black mud of the flats, beloved lair of the innkeeper worm, *Urechis caupo,* searching for its elusive burrow while my shoes slipped off because of the powerful sucking muck. At nineteen, I received a grant to study hibernation in Maltese snails. For two months I sat alone on a high stool in a damp fifty-degree cool room taking the temperatures of my sleeping snails. And it slowly dawned on me that if this was life as a research scientist, it was not for me. As my grant money ran out, taking my food money with it, I had to admit that eight weeks of shivering—and now hungry—solitude had been more than enough. I was too much of an extrovert to hole up in a lab.

So the next summer I worked as a waitress. At Calvin's Coffee Shop I had my morning regulars and loyal lunch crowd at my own six feet of counter. People seemed to feel comfortable with me right away. And I liked waiting on them in my white sneakers and my green cotton uniform with the big pocket in front for the tips. I had the salesladies from Bullocks during the lunchtime rush and in the late afternoon, the retired Filipino gardener who came in with his dead employer's dog. (The gardener had coffee; the little dog sat on the floor next to the counter stool and licked vanilla ice cream out of a Styrofoam cup cut in half). I talked to my customers and listened to the latest installments of their stories. I realized that being a waitress and being a doctor were not all that different.

So I put my tide tables and specimen jars away and decided to go into medicine.

Early on I realized that surgery wasn't a serious option for me. I was hopelessly clumsy, and I couldn't visualize anatomy in two dimensions, let alone in three. Pediatrics didn't appeal, nor did obstetrics. I tried pathology, but after ten autopsies, I wasn't sure I wanted to spend all my time with the dead. Then, during my internship, I found myself unexpectedly circling back to worms.

After a grueling night on call during which I had broken a sandal strap running up and down stairs to various emergencies, my boss told me to report to the office of the associate chief of staff for research, Dr. Lucien Guze. He wanted me to see Dr. Guze because he'd heard that when I'd called him the day before, to ask permission to use a drug in a novel way, I'd come across as surly and abrupt. What did I think I was doing treating his beloved mentor this way? I was to go over there immediately and apologize.

I walked into Dr. Guze's office with rumpled hair, grungy breath, and blood-shot eyes, punctuated by the flip-flop sound of my sandals with each step. Before I even got all the way in, I felt my right hand being warmly shaken and my whole face being embraced by the kindest pair of eyes I'd ever seen. He was a lean man in his early fifties, in a three-piece suit of light wool, looking natty and professorial at the same time. I sat down on an old leather couch near the bookshelves and Dr. Guze sat opposite me in an armchair with a low coffee table between us. He leaned forward and started getting to know me with the assurance of a man who had taken thousands of medical histories. I knew I was being deftly dissected but all I felt was a warm glow. Like my boss, Dr. Guze was an infectious disease specialist, and from that day on he was my mentor, too.

In medical school I had taken a zoologist's interest in infectious diseases, and it was the only section of my big medicine textbook I had read word for word. But in my residency I had never seriously considered the specialty because the infectious disease fellows in training at our hospital seemed so unimaginative and dull, obsessed with gathering data for clinical studies of antibiotics, and focused on tabulating every detail of blood tests and cultures. In fact, I was thinking about going into rheumatology, the study of bones, joints, and autoimmune diseases like lupus.

But when I told Dr. Guze about rheumatology he quipped, "You could learn all of rheumatology in six months." This was, of course, untrue, but I knew what he meant. In infectious diseases I would have to master both the plant and animal kingdoms, investigating a rash from the smallest virus to the infected bite of the largest lion.

He had me pegged as a worm hunter, and a year later I was studying infectious diseases under him. I learned that the free-living forms I used to study have their parasitic counterparts. The little cross-eyed planaria flatworms that grow into two-headed worms if you cut their heads in half have swarms of parasitic cousins: the liver and lung flukes, the schistosomes, and the tapeworms. The tiny free-living roundworms visible under a hand lens in a pinch of moist soil are represented in patients by the parasitic filaria, the tiny round-worms that cause elephantiasis and the intestinal ascaris worms.

And twenty years later, one of these varieties was likely causing the fevers, hives, and liver pains in my Vietnamese patient, Hanh.

Finding out where Hanh had met his worm was first a matter of retracing his steps. He had left Vietnam when he was eighteen in 1983, and now at thirty-three, he had made his first trip back. His plane landed in Ho Chi Minh City (formerly Saigon) where his uncle, aunt, and cousins met him and Vy at the airport and took them home. For four days they toured the city.

"The city was as I remembered it," Hanh told me, "the park in the middle, the Catholic basilica, the post office were all the same, only everything seemed smaller, including the people. They looked short and thin compared to us." During their four days in Ho Chi Minh City, Vy and Hanh ate traditional Vietnamese food, but everything was well cooked.

Their next stop was the old imperial capital, Hue, midway between Ho Chi Minh City and Hanoi. In addition to the usual rice and noodles, they ate land snails and crab, which are known carriers of parasitic worms. But again, all of their food was well cooked.

From Hue the couple flew to Hanoi, seven hundred miles to the north. They walked all over the city and they visited Huong, the mountain pagoda whose name means perfume. At Ha Long Bay they saw battlefields where the Vietnamese had repulsed Chinese invaders for two thousand years, and they explored the secret places where the people hid their weapons.

"Did you swim in the water there?" I asked, thinking of the fluke disease schistosomiasis.

"No, it was too cold up north to swim at that time of year."

Then they came south to the Nah Trang coast, where Hanh's uncle is a math instructor at the local college. They took a boat trip to fishing villages on nearby islands. Here Vy and Hanh ate *goi tom*, an appetizer of raw shrimp in a sweet sauce.

"Did you eat the same number of shrimp as your wife or more?" I asked.

"I ate more, and also," he added, anticipating my next question, "I went swimming there. I jumped off a boat about a mile from shore."

Finally the couple returned to Ho Chi Minh City. It was the lunar New Year. While Vy went out with her friends, Hanh's cousin, Chanh, an architect, invited him out to a farewell dinner at a restaurant that served exotic items to executives and their guests. They ate frogs, lizards, field mice, and, the *pièce de résistance*, an entire cobra. All of these dishes were deliciously seasoned and well cooked, all except the gall bladder of the cobra and its heart.

"How big was the snake?" I interrupted.

"About eight hundred grams," he replied. "That is one and a half pounds."

"The gall bladder was served raw in a little wine," he went on. "The heart was just served raw. My cousin said, 'These are for you.' I knew my brother had eaten these things during his visit, and now it was my turn."

"It was a kind of dare?" I asked.

"Yes," he replied.

I had heard about the health- and virility-enhancing powers that these cobra organs were thought to possess, but I didn't press Hanh with questions on this point. "How did they taste?"

"Pretty awful," he said.

I had gathered all my clues and I also knew the results of additional blood tests of muscle and liver. Now I had to match the m.o. of the various parasites against the particulars of Hanh's illness and come up with some likely suspects. I got out a piece of scratch paper and started making a list. I didn't waste time on the common tropical fevers, malaria and typhoid. Hanh's blood film was negative for malaria. If he had contracted typhoid he should have already responded to the antibiotics his wife had given him.

I went right to the worms because they cause the extremely high eosinophil counts, particularly if they move out of the intestines and into the tissues. Hanh didn't mention mosquito bites, but of course he and his wife were bitten. They expected to be; that's why they both took pills to prevent malaria. At least four species of filaria are transmitted by the bites of mosquitoes. Although not common in Vietnam, at least two of them may be found there. The larval roundworms pass into the host's body when the female mosquito feeds and make their way to the lymph nodes, where they mature over the next few months into white, threadlike worms that can be over an inch long. The adult worms discharge thousands of larval worms into the blood stream during the day or night to match the feeding time of local mosquitoes, and the cycle of infection between mosquito and man continues. It's the adult worms that obstruct the lymphatic system and cause the bizarre swelling of the legs (and the scrotum in males) called elephantiasis. It was possible that Hanh was suffering from the first stages of filariasis, called acute filarial fever, which the GIs got in the Pacific Theater during World War II. He had the fever and chills and high eosinophil counts that go with the syndrome, but he lacked the inflamed and painful lymph nodes that the soldiers got. It was possible that Hanh had filariasis, but it seemed unlikely.

Next I considered trichinosis, a roundworm disease contracted by eating undercooked pork. Very high eosinophil counts occur in this disease as the larval worms exit the meat, penetrate the gut, and begin migrating to the muscle of the host. But in patients as sick as Hanh was, these worms always cause enough muscle damage to elevate an enzyme called CPK. Hanh's CPK level was normal, ruling out trichinosis.

The third item on my list was schistosomiasis, the blood fluke that infects more than 200 million people worldwide. Schistosomes are quarter- to half-inch long flatworms with complex life cycles in which fresh water snails are intermediate hosts. People don't get schistosomiasis from snails directly. The infective larvae leave the snail host and burrow through the human skin of a swimmer, or a rice farmer standing in the water. Hanh had gone swimming in Vietnam, but he'd been in the ocean far enough from shore to dilute the fresh water flowing in. He probably hadn't encountered any schistosomes.

But there could've been some kind of worms in those raw shrimp Hanh and his wife had eaten on the Nah Trang coast. Here I drew a blank, although I wondered about *Paragonimus,* the lung fluke, which one catches by eating undercooked crabs and crayfish. Because of the disease caused by the lung fluke, millions of people in the Far East cough up blood, sometimes every day for years. But if Hanh had paragonimiasis he should have been coughing by now.

What I had generated so far is called a differential diagnosis, a list of disease suspects doctors make when confronted with a difficult patient. Like a detective, I was analyzing motive, means, and opportunity for each worm. But my differential diagnosis so far had left out the most important clue: Hanh was the only one on the trip who became ill; his wife and his cousins remained well. People do have varying immunity to parasites, but in this case, I suspected the answer to this patient's illness depended on the one thing he did that was different from everyone else: He ate the raw cobra. So it was time to backtrack to the snake.

I had no idea what a person could catch from eating a snake, but I suspected the answer was hiding somewhere in my office. I tipped my chair away from my cluttered desk and stared up at the pale green wall across from me, thinking. There was my children's art, a gold-framed picture of the wilds of upstate New York, my high school pencil sketch of a snail crawling up a twig, and my diplomas. And somewhere in my oak bookcase, or in my credenza bookcase, or in my ten file drawers of infectious disease articles, was Hanh's worm.

I stepped over the patient charts stacked on the floor, pulled my big infectious diseases textbook and my tropical medicine book off the shelves and laid them open on top of the stacks of lab and x-ray reports on my desk. I looked up "snake" and "cobra" in both books, but the only references were to snakes biting people, not the other way around.

Then I noticed a slim paperback book, Elaine Jong's *Travel and Tropical Medicine Manual,* which I had ordered from a catalog but had never really used. I started leafing through it, and there in the last chapter, I found exactly what I needed, a table called "Animal Helminths Commonly Transmitted to Man." Here was a list of parasitic worms that, although adapted to animal hosts, could accidentally get into people.

There was the rat lungworm, the walrus roundworm, a worm that lives in the tissues of raccoons, and there were two worms one could catch from consuming raw snake: *Spirometra,* a tapeworm, and *Gnathostoma,* a roundworm. The natural hosts of these worms were dogs, cats, and other mammals.

Spirometra causes a bizarre eye disease called sparganosis. In the Far East people put poultices of raw frog or snake muscle directly on the eye for various ailments. Tapeworm larvae then migrate from the poultice into the tissues around the eye. Eating undercooked frog or snake can also cause infection. In these cases there's fever, along with high eosinophil counts, and eventually larval tapeworms migrate from the patient's intestine into the tissues, forming tender swellings.

I skipped down the page to the paragraph on diagnosis: Wait for the nodules to form under the skin, remove one surgically, look inside for a glistening, white, slowly undulating worm. No other diagnostic tests are available. The only known treatment is surgical excision of the nodules. So *Spirometra* was a possibility, but if Hanh had this worm, there was nothing to do about diagnosis yet.

The final suspect on my list was the roundworm *Gnathostoma spinigerum*. To find out more about it, I had to turn to an old book put out by the Armed Forces Institute of Pathology titled *Pathology of Tropical and Extraordinary Diseases*. This is one of the most gruesome books in anyone's medical library, filled with photos of faces being eaten up by fungus and worms crawling across eyeballs.

In the book was a diagram of a gnathostome, anchored by its spiny head to the stomach wall of a leopard, tiger, dog, or cat. But the worm makes a circuitous journey to get there. The adult host passes eggs that are eaten by a tiny, one-eyed water bug called *Cyclops*. A fish, frog, or snake then eats the infected copepod. The larva escapes the *Cyclops* and the host's intestinal tract and forms a cyst in the muscles.

When Hanh ate the raw cobra heart, which is mostly muscle, one or more of these encysted larvae could have been liberated into his stomach by the processes of digestion. Since he wasn't a member of the dog or cat family, the larval worm would not mature to adulthood there, but instead, would burrow through his stomach wall into the abdominal cavity, penetrate the liver, and head for the muscle tissue under the skin. Hanh's symptoms fit the clinical description perfectly: fever, pain and pressure over the liver, hives, plus the highest eosinophil counts recorded in any infectious disease.

According to my book, Hanh's worm would reach the outer tissues in about a month, and then he would start to have swellings under his skin. But since man is an abnormal host for this parasite, it would not settle down in one muscle but would continue to restlessly wander through the body of the host for up to twelve years.

I read with horror that the tunneling worm sometimes finds its way into the brain. When this happens, fatal damage follows. At autopsy, worm trails zigzag the brain like they'd been made with an Etch A Sketch, and a tiny larva, still alive after the host's death, is found at the end of its last trail.

I'd gone as far as I could on my own, and now I needed to call a few experts.

Dr. Claire Panosian, at the University of California at Los Angeles, is an infectious disease doctor like me, but she studied at the famed London School of Tropical Medicine and has always had a special interest in parasitic diseases. I told her Hanh's whole story. She listened carefully, and, in her usual methodical way, she reviewed all the diagnostic possibilities, which were the same ones I'd come up with.

"You know, Pam," she added for completeness sake, "this could be eosinophilic leukemia."

"I hope not," I said, thanking her and promising to call her back with follow-up information.

I also tried Dr. Linda Croad, an infectious disease colleague at a sister facility within our HMO. Her hospital cares for a large immigrant population, so I thought she might have seen a patient like this. She agreed that the raw snake had to be the key to the diagnosis, but she didn't have any personal experience either with gnanthostomiasis or with sparganosis.

Finally, I called the Centers for Disease Control and Prevention. An operator with a friendly Georgia accent answered, "CDC, Atlanta." She connected me with Sue Partridge, a health education specialist in the parasitology branch. I identified myself as a physician infectious disease specialist, and she invited me to present Hanh's case. Ms. Partridge was impressed by Hanh's eosinophil count and thought that my roundworm diagnosis, gnathostomiasis, was a real possibility. She recommended that I consider starting therapy with the new worm medicine, albendazole.

"Do you have any blood tests for gnathostomiasis at the CDC?" I asked.

"We don't, but one of our colleagues in Thailand does," she said. "I can fax you information on how to send a specimen."

I thanked her and promised to call her with follow-up information on Hanh. Later that afternoon the fax arrived. I was directed to send two milliliters of blood at room temperature with a check for forty-five dollars via airfreight to Dr. Wanpen Chaicumpa at the faculty of tropical medicine in Bangkok. Prior notification was important because someone would have to meet the specimen at the airport and move it through customs.

After reading this, I decided to wing it and trust my hunch. Albendazole is safe and easy to take. I called Vy, told her what the experts said, and asked her to pick up the prescription for albendazole that I was going to call in to the pharmacy.

Two days later Hanh came to my clinic for an appointment. He was a lean young man with bright brown eyes and a handsome grin. We reviewed his history, and then he climbed up on the exam table. His examination was almost entirely negative, and on the surface he looked well. But he had a fast pulse, a sign of some hidden commotion. I sent him down for a repeat blood count, and his eosinophil count had climbed to an astounding twenty-five thousand. Tests for dengue fever, amebiasis, and stool parasites were negative.

But Hanh was feeling steadily better on his albendazole tablets, and his fevers were less severe every night. I ordered a literature search on gnathostomiasis from the library. Then I turned my attention to other problems.

Linda Croad called for advice about a meningitis case. She thought it might be the very contagious meningococcus. Would I suggest that she treat an entire college dormitory for possible exposure right away or wait for the culture results? Also, she wanted to know how the "cobra heart guy" was doing. A bone marrow transplant patient went into respiratory failure from pneumonia. One of my HIV patients got sick and was admitted to the hospital; another came to my clinic strung out on cocaine.

Then about two weeks later Vy called me again. "Hi, Vy," I said with a sinking feeling. "How's Hanh?"

"Oh, he's feeling much better," she said, "but he has a swelling on his abdomen for two days now."

She told me it was on his left side, was the size of a small egg, and was tender and red. So, our worm was coming to the surface and, despite two weeks of albendazole, it was still alive.

"Vy," I asked, "Do you think Hanh would agree to a minor surgical procedure? Maybe we can get rid of this worm, once and for all."

"Yes, I think he will," she said.

About a week later, I met Hanh and Vy in the minor surgery clinic. We watched while the physician's assistant anesthetized Hanh's skin and used a scalpel and scissors to remove a "two-centimeter long, very firm, non-mobile, cord-like" piece of tissue from Hanh's abdominal wall. She picked it up with forceps and dropped it into a jar of formalin. Then she closed the incision with two layers of stitches and bandaged the wound.

A few days later I went down to the basement of the hospital, and the pathologist and I, using a double-headed microscope, examined stained slides of Hanh's nodule. The tissue was filled with inflammatory cells, including the bright red eosinophils. Deep in the dermis was a tunnel of dead tissue, running through the entire specimen. The pathologist followed it from one slide to another but there was no worm, no head bulb with its four rows of spiny hooklets, no intestines, no sexual organs, no fragments of cuticle, nothing. Our quarter-inch worm had barreled a tunnel through Hanh's tissue and gone elsewhere, trailing behind it a swarm of pursuing eosinophils.

Frustrated, I stood up from the microscope feeling guilty. I had cut out a piece of my patient's body for nothing. I went to see the laboratory supervisor. It was time to send Hanh's blood to Bangkok.

As I feared, the process of sending blood to Thailand was a bureaucratic nightmare. The most difficult part was arranging for the specimen to be picked up at the Bangkok airport. Hanh had to come in twice to have his blood drawn before the lab supervisor was able to successfully make all the arrangements and get the specimen off on its journey to the other side of the world.

I had absolutely no problem getting the results, however. One afternoon a few weeks later, I was sitting at my desk at work, and an e-mail message popped up on my screen. It was from Dr. Wanpen Chaicumpa. The serum specimen sent on the patient, Hanh Le, was unequivocally positive for *Gnathostoma* by Western Blot analysis. Our diagnosis was correct.

I've since learned that a gnathostome will flee to the surface of a patient being treated with albendazole, but the worm moves so quickly that it is hard to catch. By the time doctors remove a swelling like Hanh's, the worm is usually long gone. The only exception is if a worm wanders into a dead end like a fingertip; then it is possible to remove it surgically before it has a chance to back out.

As for Hanh's worm, it just disappeared. My guess is that the albendazole killed it and that it dissolved. At any rate, after several months Hanh's eosinophil count gradually returned to normal, and he has been well ever since.

I haven't seen any more patients with gnathostomiasis yet, but I expect to someday, because the disease is not rare. A species of it occurs in Mexico and is transmitted to people through undercooked fish. Remember that when you're ordering ceviche.

Human beings live and travel all over the earth, pushing native plants and animals aside wherever they go. Because we are among the largest and most powerful animals on the planet, we forget that we can put ourselves in grave danger by not respecting the smaller creatures that are part of the natural balance, too.

When we think of natural habitats, we think of the world around us. But every animal is also the natural habitat of the creatures adapted to live inside it. When Hanh ate the snake, he evicted the spiny little worm from its red velvet house and made it a restless wanderer in an alien place.

wounded hearts

I threw the covers off and sat up.

My heart was pounding, and I felt like I was breathing in a vacuum. It was three o'clock in the morning in the call room at the Grace–New Haven Hospital in Connecticut, and in the next bed the pediatric resident was sound asleep. A big truck rattled down the highway and shook the windows of the old building. I jumped out of bed, put on my shoes, and pulled on my white lab coat. I ran down the hall, down three flights of stairs, and out of the building into the spring night.

The old houses surrounding the hospital were dark and quiet, and my lock and chain banged noisily as I unhooked my bike from the rack. I jumped on and headed for home, standing up to pump the two miles to my house as if something were after me. My white coat billowed back as I fled past houses and storefronts, across the highway bridge, past the New Haven common and its three white churches, dimly lit, on to Orange Street and finally to tree-lined Edward. In thirty minutes I was safe in my own bed on the third floor of the wooden house where I lived with two classmates.

I had abandoned my patients and run away from everything I had worked for my entire life.

I'd had an anxiety attack.

It was the clinical rotations, which started in the middle of the second year of med school, that had gradually unhinged me. Our early months had unfolded in the safe darkness of the amphitheaters, where we listened to lectures, looked at slides, and spent so much time with our one hundred classmates that we could recognize each other's silhouettes if we broke the beam of the projector.

Now, though, we were on our own. They sent us to the Fitkins, St. Raphael's, the Memorial Unit, and the Veterans Hospital in groups of two, three, or four, but for all the camaraderie I felt, I could've been alone. In the classrooms there had been no examinations and no grades, but on the wards, our friends became grim competitors for the approval of the attending physicians. The evaluations we earned from these professors determined our future: who would win the best residencies and who would enter the coveted specialties. The single-minded drive that had gotten us into medical school in the first place surged to the surface and cut us off from each other.

Most mornings I was too nervous to eat. We had to draw blood and insert IVs into sick people. When we missed they sometimes got angry, or, far worse, they quietly cried. Then you knew that you weren't a healer; you were an inept, miniature version of their disease.

By the time I got to pediatrics in the spring I was nearing the end of my rope. What should have been a benign rotation filled with jovial pediatricians and cherubic babies became, instead, a season in hell on the adolescent ward. My partner, a confident and handsome former Yale jock, would have nothing to do with me. He had reached his stride, and the attending, a dry academic with an interest in pediatric neurology, loved him. So did the nurses. He had the trim, muscular grace of a water polo player and great "hands." When he drew blood from the kids, he never seemed to miss.

I, on the other hand, was a lost soul.

Everything I saw and everything I was asked to do scared me. The residents assigned me to an eleven-year-old from South America whose chronic kidney disease had distorted the growth of all of his bones. His hands, his limbs, even his ribs were bent and dwarfed. I suffered to look at him because his disease seemed like such a terrible destiny for a child. He was just a gentle kid, but I was afraid of him—afraid of hurting him more by imposing my awkward, amateur "help" on him, and afraid of whatever it was in nature that caused such things.

The nurses could have pushed me along, as they did my golden boy partner, by asking me leading questions and by sharing their observations and jokes with me. But in those days, there was an unspoken competition between the nurses and the female med students. While they seemed to adore males, they were cool to me. They wouldn't tell me what to do, or how to do it.

So I hid out. I wandered the ward in my short white coat, tomboy khaki pants, and clunky Clark Trek shoes, helping a boy with leukemia put a few pieces into his puzzle, peeking into the microbiology lab at the end of the hall, and holing up in the call rooms or the library. The library, at least, was a legitimate place to be, because we were supposed to be studying, and I found out the South

American boy had something called "rugger jersey vertebrae." Incurable.

The culmination of this ghostly existence came the night Janine went off her rocker. She was a fourteen-year-old African-American girl from the neighborhood who had been admitted a few days before with a fever. As the medical student, I was supposed to examine Janine, write up my findings, read about her illness, and run scut. (Scut comprises miscellaneous chores that run downhill and land on the med student—drawing blood and taking it to the lab, checking results, arranging tests.) I was a poor scut runner, but I did read about Janine, who turned out to be a fascinoma from the get-go.

The word "fascinoma" is medical slang for fascinating plus "oma," usually a tumor, but here a patient. It's a case where the diagnosis is obscure and the illness is severe. With a fascinoma everyone feels that the patient has a classic case of something, but no one can figure out what it is. Janine had been on the ward for about five days with a high fever. She was a fascinoma because cultures of her blood and urine were still negative, suggesting that she didn't have an infection, and she didn't seem to have one of the fever-causing collagen diseases, like rheumatoid arthritis, either.

But Janine had a Roth spot. When we looked into her left eye with the ophthalmoscope we could see through the lens and beyond all the way to the retina, which makes up the eye's back wall. The Roth spot was a little white area set in the retina's pink field between the gold cables of the arteries and the flatter blue lines of the veins. The eye's circulatory system had hurled something there, and we could see it as a tiny point of damage, like a meteor crater.

While we were still trying to figure out where they were coming from, those same little particles in her circulatory system started
landing in her brain. I don't remember at what hour of the night
her delirium began, but I was on call. Janine was lying in bed in a
pool of light, feverish and under restraint. She was muttering and
shouting incoherently. I had no idea what to do. Her mother and
aunt, however, seemed remarkably calm and self-possessed as they
quietly read to Janine from their Bibles. I was out of the picture,
without even a diagnosis to offer. They had taken over her care.

It was that night, or maybe the next call night, that I ran away.
I was a green recruit under fire for the first time, and while I lay in
the dark of the call room, some force of self-preservation decided
to propel me all the way to California, if necessary. I know now that
it was more than just a fear of failure. It was fear of what I would
have to become to survive as a doctor. Every day I had to witness
pain, and occasionally inflict it, and the clinical rotations were a
traumatic initiation into a new way of being. I was changing forever, becoming different from people outside the world of medicine. In order to deal with suffering calmly, I was being forced to
lose my emotional response to it. The choice, as I understood it,
was to feel or to heal. And I wasn't sure who I'd be if I chose the
path of healing over the fullness of feeling.

Yale Med wasn't unaware of what it was asking of us, and it
dealt with my crisis gently. Everyone knows how hard it is to get
into medical school, but few people realize how loath a school is to
throw you out once you get there. I think the administrators saw us
as high-strung thoroughbreds, skittish at the starting gate, but potentially fast as hell on the track. They gave one particularly brilliant

student, my future husband, Glenn, a stereo system to cheer him up. They assigned me to a female psychiatric resident.

Dr. Slatkin had gone into medicine after having a family and was just the right person to take me in hand. She offered me heavy-duty tranquilizers, but I opted instead for three days off and a series of appointments with her, at Yale's expense. I spent those three days wandering over the New Haven green taking black-and-white pictures of sleeping drunks. They were outsiders like me, but they seemed oblivious to failure.

I recovered my nerve and went back to the hospital. I finished pediatrics and went on to neurosurgery, where I poked needles into the unanesthetized radial arteries of women with bone metastases from breast cancer.

"Why do you have to do this, Doctor?" frightened women whispered through their tears. I myself wasn't clear on the reason for the test. I only knew why *I* was doing it: because the resident told me to.

I held back livers with retractors until my arm ached, while the surgeon removed the patient's gall bladder. I scrubbed in on six-hour heart surgeries, at the end of which the patient's heart couldn't be restarted no matter how many times we made it jump with the paddles. I was completely overwhelmed the first two times I walked into surgery, and I backed out of the room as quickly as I entered to avoid throwing up in my mask.

Nowadays, medical students are offered much more emotional support than when I was going through these early clinical rotations in 1973. Back then many of us were trained by doctors who believed that our survival depended on our ability to lead with our heads instead of our hearts. A disconnect between facts and feelings was seared into us, sometimes in a most brutal way. During one of my early clinical rotations, the senior resident paged me to the bedside of the patient I was taking care of at the VA. The old man, whom I had been talking to a few hours earlier, was dying, and the resident wanted me to see the agonal heart rhythms on the monitor. But I arrived a moment too late; Emil had just gone flat line. I stood behind the resident looking at the pale soles of that nice old man's feet.

"Ah, there you are!" the resident said, turning around. "You just missed an interesting heart rhythm. Maybe I can get him to do it again," he said, striking Emil's skinny chest with the flat part of his fist. But the green line stayed flat. "Too bad," he said and walked off. I just stood there feeling like a fool because nobody had told me that my patient was going to die. I looked around to make sure the resident was gone. Then I put my hand on his cooling chest and said, "Goodbye, Emil."

By the time I got to the abortion clinic and stood at the stir-rup end of the procedure, I was numb to almost everything. But it was in this clinic that I found out that my numbness was not yet covered by emotional insulation, a toughening process that would come later. My actual state was one of openness and vulnerability, and because of this a ray of light from an unexpected source was about to pierce my soul.

The neighborhood teenagers climbed up on the table in hospital gowns open in the back with a sheet wrapped around their waists. There was a flash of red in the suction tube, a yelp, and then they climbed down white-faced and shaky while the resident said,

"Next." There was nothing for me to do but watch. Idly I turned around and looked down into one of the vacuum bottles.

At first all I saw was a pool of red and yellow glup. Then, as I was about to turn away, I saw a tiny hand that had been torn free. The light from the overhead surgical lamp shone through each pale pink finger. At first I just stood frozen. Then suddenly I was shot through and through with a joyful awe. In that moment, all of my fear and anxiety about my suitability as a doctor, my concern about the numbness that was stealing my sense of compassion, the emotional confusion and feelings of insecurity that had so troubled me during the past year, all seemed to make a strange kind of sense in that one moment. In those tiny translucent fingers, I knew for certain that what I was seeing was the hand of God. And it wasn't pointing at me or accusing me. It was reaching up past me toward something over my right shoulder from which it could not be separated.

Although I have never been formally religious, the vivid memory of this experience has never faded. Since then I have always been able to feel the spiritual side of things and to believe in divine and invisible powers. It was only by touching bottom in the weeks that proceeded that afternoon that I able to see something much higher as well. Like Moses, who hid himself in the cleft of the rock, I was allowed a glimpse of something radiant. It was what I got in exchange for what I was losing.

What I lost as a result of all of my experiences that year was part of my emotional range. Since then I've never been able to cry in front of anyone who isn't a family member. But as a result of my training, I do have equanimity; I'm cool under fire. My feelings never make me panic or run away anymore, no matter how hopeless or depressing the patient's illness is.

As for Janine, my fascinoma, whose mysterious ailment was the beginning of the transformation of my too-open heart, I'll never forget that her perplexing illness was finally traced back to her heart, as well. Just before I left the adolescent ward, there appeared in her blood cultures a tiny rod-shaped bacillus called by the fanciful and rhyming name *Haemophilus aphrophilus,* pronounced with the accent on the second syllable of each word. It's a relatively rare cause of infectious endocarditis, the term for an infection inside the heart, usually on a valve. I've only seen a few cases since. Luckily, the microbiology professor in the lab at the end of the hall had been one of the first researchers to describe the organism. Otherwise, with the technology available then, they might not have been able to grow this germ, which will not appear unless its special requirements are met.

The residents started Janine on antibiotics, and her life was saved. However, toward the end of my last year in medical school I found out at what price. I was taking an elective in electrocardiogram interpretation in children. Another senior student and I were sitting in a small room with the instructor, a renowned pediatric cardiologist. Each of us was going through a stack of EKGs. I picked up the next tracing and there was Janine Jackson's name in the upper left-hand corner. She was now sixteen. The EKG looked OK, so I turned to the professor and asked, "Whatever happened to this patient?"

"Janine? Oh, she wound up having her aortic valve replaced," she answered.

So Janine had had an infected aortic valve. "That's bad," I thought. "She'll grow out of the valve they put in, and they'll have to open her chest and put a bigger one in, or at the very least replace this one when it wears out. And all her life she'll be at risk for infection on her new valve."

A short time later, I graduated and headed back to California with an M.D. after my name. Even before I specialized in infectious diseases, there were always patients with infectious endocarditis. Imperfections of the heart, like leaky or tight valves, are surprisingly common. One in a hundred babies is born with some cardiac abnormality. Each defect, whether congenital or acquired, as in rheumatic fever, makes the owner vulnerable to heart infection.

When I put my stethoscope to a person's chest what I'm listening for are signs of the heart's flaws. In a normal adult heart, all you hear are the sounds of the heart valves snapping shut after the blood flows across them. The blood's flow, as it moves across normal heart valves and around cardiac structures that are smooth and without abnormal perforations, is smooth and silent. It's called laminar flow, the same quiet, unbroken stream you get if you turn on a faucet just a little. If the edge of a heart valve is rough with scar or calcium, the aperture is leaky or fused shut, or there is a hole in a septum of the heart, the blood will flow through with a whoosh. This is turbulent flow, and it's also what happens across a water faucet that is clogged or opened wide. When doctors hear a murmur, they're hearing turbulent flow across something abnormal in the heart.

That's important because it's one of the factors that open the door to heart infections. Turbulent flow causes wear and tear on the heart's delicate lining, and damaged lining is sticky for platelets. Platelets, in turn, are sticky for bacteria, which cause endocarditis. Are there bacteria circulating in the blood stream? You bet. Every time you use dental floss or even chew on something hard, bacteria living between the teeth may be propelled into the blood. Even more alarming is the fact that a trip to your dentist for a simple cleaning can send enough bacteria into your circulation to detect with routine blood cultures. Bacteria slip over normal valves, but they stick to platelets on valves or other heart structures that are subject to turbulent flow.

As the bacteria multiply and begin to do their damage, you probably won't feel a thing. The outside of the heart hurts like a skinned knee if it's inflamed, but the heart valves, where most cases of endocarditis occur, rarely register pain. So infectious endocarditis is often a devious disease, making its presence known by indirect signs like Janine's Roth spot and particular rashes.

One of my professors in medical school told me a story about a medical student who lived in the days before antibiotics. He had a leaky aortic valve, and because so much blood had to be ejected by the heart to get some of it forward into his circulation, he could feel each pulse pound in his head. He knew that he was not going to live a normal life span; either his overworked heart would fail or his damaged aortic valve would get infected. And in those days, an infected heart valve was a death sentence.

One summer evening he was leaving his sister's house where he'd been studying, and as he pulled on his coat, he saw a cluster of maroon spots, called petechiae, under the skin of his palm. Recognizing these spots as the rash of endocarditis, he turned to his sister and said, "I shall be dead by Christmas." And, despite everything that could be done for him, he was right.

But even a normal heart valve can get infected if enough bacteria are injected into the blood stream. And users of intravenous drugs do this to themselves every day. The heroin or crack they inject is often contaminated, and if the drugs themselves aren't, the liquid they're dissolved in—tap water, saliva, or even toilet bowl water—often is. Sometimes the bacteria on the user's own skin find their way in with the needle.

Most often, intravenous drug abusers infect the tricuspid valve on the right side of the heart. This valve is the least essential because it guards the portal to the low-pressure side of the circulation, the part that leads to the lungs. However, for unknown reasons, a virulent organism, *Staphylococcus aureus*, commonly infects this valve in drug users. When they come to the hospital they appear to have pneumonia because infection travels from the tricuspid valve downstream to both lungs. It's more than pneumonia, and experienced doctors aren't fooled when they see the fever and the brown scarred veins of the patient.

"How long have you been sick?" they ask.

"I don't know, about a week, maybe," the patient answers.

"When did you last fix?"

"About three months ago," comes the unreliable reply.

If they stay in the hospital long enough, these patients usually get well with intravenous antibiotics. Sometimes their friends make their hospital time more bearable by sneaking in drugs for them to use through their convenient intravenous line.

If endocarditis destroys the tricuspid valve, we usually don't have to replace it. But when the infection attacks the vital aortic valve that controls blood flow to the high-pressure side of the circulation, the patient needs a new one—even if he or she can't get off drugs.

I remember a man at the Veterans Hospital who was only in his twenties when he had his aortic valve replaced after it had been damaged by endocarditis following heroin abuse. We hoped he would kick his habit through the VA drug treatment program.

Then one afternoon he came in for the last time. I was working in the emergency room. At first glance the problem had nothing to do with his heart. He was in agony, grasping his left leg in both hands. Blurry tattoos covered the old tracks on his skinny arms. His leg was cold and blue. He was too young to have circulatory problems from hardening of the arteries. My guess was an acute embolus, a big clot from his new heart valve, which was probably infected.

"Jimmy, have you been using again?" I asked.

"No, I swear," he answered. And maybe he was telling the truth. A prosthetic aortic valve can get infected spontaneously.

We saved his leg but we couldn't save his life. The surgeons opened the femoral artery and removed a worm-shaped clot that had blocked it completely. The clot was packed with the yeast *Candida albicans,* the same fungus that causes vaginal infections. When it infects a heart valve, it's impossible to eradicate with antibiotics alone. The surgeons had to replace Jimmy's prosthetic aortic valve with a new one. But the new valve got infected with the same hink. At any rate Jimmy didn't survive. A patient only gets a few chances with endocarditis; after that it's a losing battle.

Since then I've treated hundreds of patients with infective endocarditis. Now we have cardiac echo machines that can find even small clumps of bacteria, platelets, and clots hanging off a heart valve. These masses, called vegetations, are the hallmark of the disease. They fly back and forth across the valve, breaking into fragments that are carried by the blood to skin, artery, or brain.

The cardiologist can even pass an ultrasensitive probe into the patient's esophagus and get right up against the back of the heart for an inside view. The transesophageal echocardiogram, as it's called, is the best way to evaluate infected prosthetic heart valves. The bacteria or fungi tend to eat around the sewing ring, loosening it stitch by stitch. When we manage these patients, the cardiologist and I want to know whether the valve is still stable, or if it's starting to rock loose and leak. I heard that one of my former patients was found dead in the bathroom with his prosthetic aortic valve upstream in an artery in his neck. Now that we have better echo techniques, we can get these patients to cardiac surgery before that happens.

The echo test lets us see the crime, but the microbiology lab nabs the criminal, the causative germ. Once it grows, I order tests of its sensitivity or resistance to various antibiotics to find the drug or drug combinations that have the best chance of sterilizing the vegetation. This is because the germ-fighting cells in the circulating blood can't penetrate these dense structures and kill the bacteria inside. Instead, the antibiotics have to get in and kill them. And since the patient will need to be treated anywhere from two to six weeks, I have to find the safest antibiotic combination.

"Safest" sometimes means the combination of drugs that will do the least damage. An elderly patient of mine, who liked to listen to music tapes in the hospital, had a resistant infection on his prosthetic mitral valve. His heart was not strong enough to tolerate another valve surgery, so I said, "I'll do my best to cure you with antibiotics. But I want you to understand that you'll probably lose some hearing as a result of the treatment." He told me to go ahead. The pharmacists dosed the drugs carefully and checked the blood levels and, fortunately, the infection cleared with only a little hearing loss. He could just as easily have gone deaf and still needed surgery. Dosing patients like him and knowing the risks is always a judgment call based on my experience with all the Janines and Jimmys I have watched suffer with endocarditis.

I have been treating patients with infectious endocarditis continuously since my earliest medical student days. By remembering these patients with their wounded hearts, I can trace my own emotional and spiritual evolution as a physician. I can glimpse what I once was before my training irrevocably wounded my own heart. I can accept the clinical calmness I have and use every day, even though I know I lack emotions that other people take for granted. And though other memories fade, I have kept bright that terrible afternoon in the abortion clinic when I was startled by the presence of God.

Even before I read Henri J. M. Nouwen's book, *The Wounded Healer*, I knew I was a wounded healer. As a Jewish person, I especially remember one story in it from the Talmud:

Rabbi Yoshua ben Levi came upon Elijah the prophet . . .

He asked Elijah, "When will the Messiah come?"

Elijah replied:

"Go and ask him yourself."

"Where is he?"

"Sitting at the gates of the city."

"How shall I know him?"

"He is sitting among the poor covered with wounds. The others unbind all their wounds at the same time and then bind them up again. But he unbinds one at a time and binds it up again, saying to himself, 'Perhaps I shall be needed: if so I must always be ready so as not to delay for a moment.'"

I still don't understand the purpose of the suffering I've seen, but I have come to believe that I'm supposed to witness it so I can help the next patient. When I was very young I fled through the gates of the city but I didn't find the Messiah. I came back and learned and healed by wounding, and that wounded me. Then one day, all alone in a room full of people, and under glaring lights, I caught a glimpse of God. And God, I saw, was suffering, too.

valley fever

Roger's funeral took place north of Los Angeles in Santa Clarita on a hot August afternoon in 1997. I sat next to his father, Jack, in the cemetery chapel. Roger's mother had died several years before. This big man, now crammed into a tight black suit, had become so close to me in the five years I had cared for his son that I felt like his daughter. I remembered how Jack and I had crouched over Roger as he lay on his side for one of his spinal taps. While I guided the long needle between the bones in his son's back, Jack had held Roger by the arms and legs, helping him curl himself up in a tight ball so I could get in. Our faces had almost touched as we bent over the stricken man.

I had put Jack through a lot trying to save his son but I'd been defeated in the end by a tiny fungus, *Coccidioides immitis*, "cocci" (pronounced KOK-see) for short.

Cocci doesn't cause funerals in Paris, Tokyo, or Cairo because the fungus grows only in the soil of the Western Hemisphere. In the American Southwest, it flourishes in the Lower Sonoran Life Zone, the dry lands of creosote and mesquite, kangaroo rats and the long-eared desert fox. Before imported water turned stretches of its habitat into farmland and suburbs, cocci thrived with little consequence to humans. But development has landed about four million of us Lower Sonorans squarely in the midst of areas where the concentration of cocci organisms in the soil is high, and the risk of acquiring cocci is great.

In general, people do not catch cocci from each other. It's an infectious disease, but not a contagious one. You get cocci by breathing in the spores that the fungus produces in the soil, and in cocci country, practically anything that disturbs the dry land, releasing the spores, can lead to infection—construction, an earthquake, an archaeological dig, dirt-biking, dust storms. The strong winds that blow in Southern California every year between Thanksgiving and Christmas are harbingers of the cocci cases we see in the following months. Wind fills the air with tiny, barrel-shaped arthrospores that, when inhaled, take up residence in the lungs, where they become round cells that grow and multiply. In about a half to two-thirds of those who encounter cocci, the presence of the fungus in the lungs might pass unnoticed, or feel like a cold or the flu, with symptoms of fever, coughing, body aches, and fatigue. And generally, that one insignificant brush with the fungus is it—it makes us immune to cocci.

But for a small percentage of people, especially those with weakened immune systems, cocci becomes a lifelong, life-changing companion. High on the list are people with HIV, Filipino or African-American men, and women in their third trimester of pregnancy (whose immune functions are reduced to keep the body from treating the fetus as a foreign object). What felt like a cold to someone else might for them turn into severe pneumonia or a treatable, but not curable, meningitis. It's cocci pneumonia that walks in Southern California hospital doors every December and January, and cocci meningitis that I've always dreaded seeing in patients like Roger. Before the advent of AIDS, cocci meningitis was the worst chronic condition that infectious disease specialists in southern California had to treat, and for many years it was almost always fatal.

Since the disease is not widely publicized, many people are unaware that cocci infects one hundred thousand new patients in the Southwest every year. And if you've heard of it at all, chances are it's only because you live in one of the cocci hotspots: Tucson and Phoenix, Arizona; Bakersfield, California; or California's San Joaquin Valley, which gave the disease its common name, Valley Fever.

As it happens, the hospital where I work is about a mile from a onetime Southern California cocci zone, Canoga Park (now paved over enough to be safer), and many of our patients live in another currently hot area, Simi Valley. (It's a given that a chronic pneumonia patient from Simi Valley who comes in after the winter winds has cocci until proven otherwise.) Infectious disease doctors in cocci country cut their teeth on the disease, and I grew up with it as a doctor. I've lived with my patients as they endured the disease and the treatments that sometimes killed them, and I've come closer to some of them, over our years together, than to many of the other people I treat. I've lost a good share of patients to all kinds of diseases, but I've only gone to four patients' funerals in my years of practice, and two of them were for young men with cocci.

Cocci can take its victims quickly. In December of 1992, following unusually heavy winds, a thirty-five-year-old Filipino man came to our hospital with Valley Fever pneumonia in both lungs. At first he seemed to rally with treatment; but after a few days it was clear that his infection was overwhelming him. I remember him sitting on the edge of his bed, naked from the waist up, his chest heaving under his smooth brown skin, his eyes opened wide, with a wild look like a frightened horse.

Dr. Hans Einstein, the grand old man of cocci, who practiced until his retirement at the Bakersfield Memorial Hospital, right in the cocci epicenter, had been helping me with the case by telephone. Hans has been tracking and treating cocci for years, and he's the co-author of such notable articles as 1978's "Tempest from Tehachapi Takes Toll or Coccidioides Conveyed Aloft and Afar," which he wrote with another great cocci expert, Demosthenes Pappagianis, the man in charge of the Coccidioidomycosis Serology Laboratory at the University of California at Davis for the past thirty years.

The 1978 report began: "To the exports from Bakersfield, California, and environs—oil, livestock, cotton, potatoes, grapes, Merle Haggard, Buck Owens—can be added one of dubious value, coccidioidomycosis." The tempest referred to in the title was a severe dust storm that "blew through Kern County on December 20, 1977." Soil carried by the storm was observed from the northern and coastal areas of San Francisco to as far north as Oregon, and in twelve weeks there were 532 cases of acute cocci, along with reports of several dogs that became ill and a gorilla in the San Francisco Zoo that died of the disease. The intimacy with a disease that comes from dealing with such epidemics was what I had hoped to tap in consulting with Dr. Einstein.

When he came to Los Angeles to visit his family for the holidays, Dr. Einstein made a special trip out to the San Fernando

Valley, at no charge to anyone. He and I sat down with this patient's parents, his pregnant wife, the pastor of his church, and other family members. The patient's three-year-old son tried to dash past us into the ICU to be with his father; an uncle stopped him as he was about to leap through the double doors of the unit.

Dr. Einstein became compassionately involved in this all too familiar tragedy. I watched his kind old face as he explained that the young man was going to die of pneumonia because a fungus in his lungs was multiplying too fast and causing too much damage for any known treatment to stop it.

Over the next few days, my patient's lungs filled with fluid and fungal cells. We dialed up the oxygen to 100 percent and backed each breath with high pressure trying to drive the oxygen into his blood stream. He hung on for a few more days but finally the weakened walls of both his lungs ruptured, and we lost him.

In that same terrible month, a young woman arrived in labor. She delivered a healthy baby, but her lungs and placenta were riddled with cocci. After the delivery she looked at her child briefly, then her breathing failed and the doctors had to put her on the ventilator as well. There was nothing anyone could do to stop the fungus or the damage it was causing. We had seen the worst that cocci could do to a human being.

In the earliest days, cocci was thought to be uniformly fatal, because all of the early patients who came to medical attention eventually died. From 1892, when it was first described in the tissues of a soldier in Argentina, through the 1920s, the diagnosis was regarded as a death sentence. But in 1929, a medical student named Chope, who was working with cocci in the laboratory, opened a culture plate containing the cottony, gray colonies. He accidentally inhaled a cloud of arthrospores and eight days later, came down with fever and pneumonia.

"Chope was heralded worldwide as a martyr to science," relates Dr. David Stevens in the fourth edition of Mandell's *Principles and Practice of Infectious Diseases*. University officials felt responsible for the tragedy and sent the young student to a sanitorium in Arizona, all expenses paid. Contrary to expectations, however, Chope made a complete recovery in a few weeks. Today, like Chope, most patients afflicted with cocci recover without medical treatment.

But when they don't, what may be years of monitoring and battling the disease begin. With cocci, there's no mysterious worm to find or identify, no puzzling symptoms waiting for a crackerjack diagnosis. Most often, the art of doctoring in serious cocci cases is in figuring out exactly what the patients' likely destiny is going to be with a disease that may be with them for life. If they have pneumonia, how likely are they to clear the infection without treatment; what is their risk of relapse in the lung or of it spreading to the skin, bone, or brain?

I remember one African-American mailman who developed cocci pneumonia in the winter of 1978. He reported to the laboratory every month for tests to measure the cocci antibodies in his blood, and at first, he seemed to be recovering well. Then, three months after the beginning of his illness, the antibodies in his blood began to rise. I asked him to come in and see me on the infectious diseases ward at the Veterans Administration Hospital in West Los Angeles, where I was working as a medical resident.

"How are you feeling?" I asked.

"OK, Doc, except for this back pain."

He took off his shirt, and I listened to his lungs. From the outside he looked fit enough, though he moved gingerly because of his
tender back. I found a hard rubber reflex hammer and struck each of
his vertebrae in turn. When I got to about the fourth thoracic, he
jumped. A bone scan confirmed that the cocci infection had invaded
the bones of his spine. He recovered after several months of treatment. His cocci was limited to his lung and his spine.

Sometimes, cocci spreads to the skin and nowhere else. A
friend of mine, who was a particularly bright surgical resident, was
performing a sigmoidoscopy on a Hispanic patient, also at the VA.

"I get the scope up the guy's rectum," he told me, "when I see
this weird crusty bump on his rear end. So I took a biopsy and
what do you think? Cocci!"

We could never find any evidence of more serious infection
elsewhere in this patient, and the same was true of a recent patient of
mine, whose cocci appeared only at the top edge of his right ear lobe.

The most dreaded complication of all is cocci meningitis,
which develops most often in young men, Caucasians included. In
meningitis the fungus finds its way into the central nervous system
and multiplies in the fluid that surrounds the brain inside and out.
There are no mild cases of this disease. Even today it is considered
incurable, and back then, almost all of the patients afflicted with
cocci meningitis eventually died from it. The lining of the brain reacts to the multiplying fungus with inflammation, and, as Hans
Einstein writes in one of his articles, "A shaggy, thickened membrane is seen at the base of the brain." This membrane blocks the
flow of cerebrospinal fluid where it leaves the brain on its way to the
spinal column. Fluid then collects under high pressure inside the

brain, a condition called obstructive hydrocephalus. When patients develop obstructive hydrocephalus, the neurosurgeon must immediately route the fluid past the block with a shunt or the patient will slip into a coma and die.

Until the late 1980s, a unique antibiotic, amphotericin B, nicknamed "amphoterrible" was the only effective treatment for severe infections caused by *Coccidioides immitis*. It poisons fungi by punching holes in their outer cell membranes, but it is poisonous to human cells as well. The kidney and the blood-forming factory in the bone marrow are especially sensitive. Patients who receive a full course of amphotericin almost always develop some kidney damage and anemia, so we minimize the damage by giving the drug in small doses over several months. And in the best cases, the side effects disappear over time.

But long-term effects are only part of the picture. The drug has some nasty immediate effects as well—chills, fever, and rapid breathing—that peak at about thirty minutes and take two to four hours to subside. One patient told me, "I was shaking so hard, I couldn't even breathe!" Nausea and vomiting are also common, so before giving amphotericin B, we also give medications to prevent pain and fever. (Recently, less toxic preparations of the drug have become available.)

Side effects aside, the drug has one more serious drawback: It does not move from the blood into the brain and has to be introduced directly into the central nervous system, which is no easy task.

The central nervous system is a fortress. A leathery membrane, the dura mater, surrounds the soft structures of the brain and spinal cord, and the dura itself is encased by the bones of the skull and spine. In order to introduce medicine into the space below the dura, the central nervous system, it is necessary to breach these defenses with a long needle. The easiest place to gain access is between the bones in the small of the back, below the level at which the spinal cord ends. Even then, the patient, who is usually lying on his side, has to curl up into the tightest possible ball to open up a little gap between the spines of the backbone. Only then can a needle be passed between these spines into the space that contains the cerebrospinal fluid. This procedure is the same as a lumbar puncture or spinal tap, but instead of taking fluid out for tests, we squirt the amphotericin B in with a syringe.

The problem with introducing the medicine there is that cerebrospinal fluid flows downhill, and the medication tends to stay where it is injected, never reaching the infected parts of the brain higher up. The drug is also highly irritating; it turns the fluid in the lower back from a clear watery solution into a thick, yellow liquid resembling motor oil. Patients could be kept alive if they got these treatments two or three times a week, but within months to a few years, they would have to be stopped. Irritation to the nerve roots would give the patient intolerable leg pains, or the space would become closed up with scar tissue.

By 1978, we were trying other ways of introducing amphotericin B into the brain. I was a first year medical resident, having survived my harrowing year as an intern, and was finally coming into my own as a doctor. The infectious disease ward was a small unit with about fifteen beds. I was the junior resident, and I had one intern under me, Dave, a slightly irreverent person with long straight brown hair, a direct brown-eyed gaze, and a raffish grin.

Two outpatients with cocci meningitis came to our infectious disease ward. One patient was a quiet African-American man in his fifties who took the bus from downtown, a ride of over an hour. The other patient, George, was a Caucasian man in his late twenties who worked in the hospital cafeteria and came up to the ward for care. He always had a cheerful "Hello" for us when we went down for lunch. He was handsome, with a soldier's bearing.

For these men, the best treatment we could offer was another new and painful way to administer their amphotericin. Since the infection is always most severe at the base of the brain where the skull meets the neck, the attending physicians decided to try injecting in the neck, instead of the lower spine, and that meant that each new resident who came on the ward learned how to do lateral cervical punctures. With the patient lying motionless on his back and looking up at the ceiling, we slowly inserted a long spinal needle just behind the ear. If the needle was inserted in exactly the right spot, it could be pushed between the bones of the spine, through the ligaments of the neck and the dura mater all the way to the base of the brain where it joins the spinal cord. Once in, we attached a syringe with amphotericin B to the needle and slowly injected the medicine into the space around the base of the brain.

That's how the procedure went in theory. In practice, though, it was all too easy to push the needle in a millimeter too far. Then the patient got ghastly electric pains down his legs and could suffer damage, paralysis, or even death. (Remember the pithed frogs in biology class?)

In medical training, we have an adage, "See one, do one, teach one." The attending physician on the infectious disease service walked me through the procedure once, and after that I was on my own. Today, such a procedure would be done with the guidance of fluoroscopic x-ray, which shows the position of the needle in rela-tion to the patient's spine. But then it was done blindly, in a small room on the ward. The needle was very thin and I do not remem-ber using any local anesthesia. As I advanced it through the layers of muscle and the membranes around the spinal cord, I could feel a series of popping sensations when I got close to the right place. Inside the needle, a long wire called a stylet filled the cavity so the needle wouldn't get clogged with tissue as it was pushed in. Each time I felt a pop, I would pull out the stylet and wait to see a trickle of cerebrospinal fluid emerge from the open end of the needle. Sometimes the patient would whisper with the last little pop, "I think you're in, Doc."

Each man received two treatments a week, so a resident rotat-ing through the infectious disease ward for a month was responsi-ble for giving sixteen treatments in all.

Medical procedures are not really my thing. I'm not that good with my hands, and I would have much preferred that Dave did the punctures. But, as an intern, he was not yet a licensed physician. I, on the other hand, had had my medical license for six months. I prepared for my injection days by skipping my usual cup of coffee, my way of ensuring that I'd have steady hands. And it was remark-able, my neuroradiology colleagues jokingly tell me today, that I got through my month's tour on the ward without paralyzing anyone.

The successor I trained was not so lucky. One afternoon after a treatment, the patient who lived downtown collapsed on his bus ride home and could not move. The injection had probably damaged a small blood vessel, and the accumulation of blood in the spinal cord caused temporary paralysis an hour or so after the procedure.

Ultimately, the lateral cervical punctures failed, at least for these two patients. Both died of complications of their cocci meningitis within a few years.

Infectious disease specialists kept looking for a safer way to use amphotericin B with cocci meningitis patients, and many began to try a technique that let them give the drug directly into the brain. They did this by implanting Ommaya reservoirs. Developed in the mid-1960s by a neurosurgeon of that name, the reservoir is a rubber balloon, about the size of a grape, connected to a small plastic tube. The neurosurgeon inserts the device under the skin over the right side of the skull. He drills a small hole through the underlying bone, and pokes the plastic tube through the hole and adjacent brain into the fluid-filled cavity inside, called the right ventricle of the brain. The scalp hair growing over the Ommaya reservoir is kept short by clipping and shaving. Before each injection, the scalp over the Ommaya is cleaned with iodine solution and alcohol. Then the rubber balloon under the skin is punctured with a small needle connected to a syringe of amphotericin B. The medicine is gradually introduced over a few minutes.

The treatment has to be started slowly, with minute doses of the drug that are increased over several weeks so the patient can become accustomed to it. But despite these precautions, patients often develop nausea shortly after the injection. One patient used to come to the infectious disease clinic at Harbor UCLA Medical Center twice a week for amphotericin B injections through his Ommaya, getting his treatments from a series of infectious disease fellows through the years. He was a man in his late twenties, with black hair cut short. He had the usual little bulge on the right side of his skull where the device was implanted. "Hi, Doc," he would say with a smile as I came through the door of the examination room, and then he would promptly vomit into an emesis basin. It was a conditioned reflex, brought on by seeing any physician coming toward him with a syringe of amphotericin B.

Another patient who received injections from all the fellows in infectious diseases was Kenji, a Japanese-American man in his early thirties. In his years of living with cocci meningitis, he'd received each new "state of the art" treatment, moving from lumbar injections, which inflamed his nerves, to an Ommaya reservoir. His brain was more tolerant of amphotericin B than his lumbar spine had been. He used to come once or twice a week to the infectious diseases laboratory building at Harbor General, sitting in a chair while we trimmed the hair around the Ommaya. He was a slight man who already had a few white hairs among the black. He would talk about his girlfriend, his work, and his skiing trips. Unless we asked him, he didn't talk about the pain in his legs from the amphotericin injections he had had in his back. For a long time he did fairly well, but in the end, it was the Ommaya, itself, that killed him. He developed a chronic infection from the device, complicated by bleeding into the brain, and six years after he'd encountered cocci, he slipped into a coma and never woke up. His was my first cocci funeral.

I had been at my HMO for three years when I met Roger. I considered myself a seasoned veteran of the cocci wars, but I will never forget how he looked that night. He was sitting on the edge of his hospital bed holding his head in his hands and rocking back and forth with pain. He had been vomiting for several days, and there was a partly filled emesis basin on the bedside table.

"My head feels like it's going to explode," he said.

Roger's troubles had started almost a year before, in 1991. He was twenty-eight, a postal worker, and had been admitted to another hospital with meningitis. He'd had high fever, confusion, and a cut on his forehead from falling. Roger's doctor treated him with antibiotics, and he seemed to improve, although no specific bacteria were ever cultured from his cerebrospinal fluid. His headache got better and his thinking cleared, and he was discharged to the house he shared with his father and his pet cats. He returned to work at the post office.

Occasionally, he would have a mild headache, but in September of the following year, he came back to his doctor with a more severe headache and a stiff neck. After that, his headaches got progressively worse. On the Friday afternoon in early October 1992 when Roger came to the hospital clutching his head, I was almost certain, based on his history, that he had cocci, because cocci is one of the few forms of meningitis that can smolder for a whole year without killing the patient.

Roger was short, with already thinning light brown hair and a soft voice; his expression was open and innocent. I told him we were going to do an operation and make his headache go away. As he looked at me with trust and relief, I held back from telling him about his cocci future. I knew he and I would be together until the end of his life.

Roger's father stood anxiously at the bedside looking at his only child. Jack was much bigger and heavier than his son, bald on top with gray-brown hair on the sides. He had a ruddy face and was, despite his size, not at all intimidating. In fact, both of these men had the same gentle eyes, like biblical shepherds. Jack listened without interrupting when I explained that his son probably had chronic meningitis due to Valley Fever. "There's a dangerous build up of pressure inside Roger's brain, and the neurosurgeon is going to insert a shunt to relieve it," I told them. "After your surgery," I added, "we will start the medical treatment for your cocci meningitis." I did not go into details yet; Roger was too sick and Jack was too upset to absorb the information.

The neurosurgeon, Dr. Farhad Arian, explained to Roger how he would put a little tube into the right ventricle of the brain and connect it to a longer tube, which he would insert under the skin behind the ear. "This tube will continue down the side of your neck and under the skin of your chest. It will empty inside the abdominal cavity, so that the excess fluid can drain freely."

Roger had to have the shunt, but it would definitely complicate his cocci treatment. It wouldn't be possible to inject amphotericin into his right ventricle through an Ommaya reservoir. All of the medicine would go straight out through the shunt tubing and into his abdominal cavity. None of it would get to the site of active infection at the base of his brain because the openings there were blocked.

I was thinking about all this as I left Roger and his father and returned to my office to pick up my briefcase so I could head home. I was exhausted and in the midst of my own drama. Daniel Lerner, a close friend and one of my two partners in infectious diseases, had died three months before, and the section chief, Debra Sachs, was out with a difficult pregnancy. I was at the halfway mark of being the sole infectious disease specialist—on call 24/7—for six intense months.

I'm fortunate to have kept a journal during this hectic time. The next day, Glenn took our six-year-old daughter, Ellen, to get her first haircut. I remember going to check on Roger. The shunt surgery had gone well, and he was feeling much better, except for a sore chest where the tube had been burrowed under his skin. I finished my rounds by lunchtime and drove the seven miles down the Ventura Freeway home. We went to a Thai place in Northridge for lunch and then across the street to an electronics store where I bought my first cell phone, a big gray Motorola. Then we went to an aquarium store and bought a tank and seven fish. Six fish were all that Ellen felt she could be responsible for, so the seventh, Zeebee, was assigned to me. Memories overlap that way—the hospital, home, hospital, home. Roger was vivid to me from the beginning because he was facing an infection that was both life-threatening and chronic.

Roger went home to his dad and his cats. The next week we put in a permanent intravenous line near his collarbone and started an arduous two-month course of amphotericin B. Each treatment took half a day, and Roger suffered from all of the usual side effects. It was important to keep the cocci from popping up somewhere else in his body, like his bones.

I wasn't sure what to do with Roger's meningitis so I called Dr. Einstein in Bakersfield. "Hans, I've got a young man here with Valley Fever meningitis and hydrocephalus. What should I do?" I remember his sympathetic groan at the other end of the line.

I decided that the best treatment would be to inject the amphotericin directly around the base of the brain, as I had done years ago during my residency. But now I had the expert help of two neuroradiologists, who would give the injections twice a week with the aid of fluoroscopic x-ray. Instead of going in from the side, they planned to inject Roger at the point where the back of his head met his neck. This is called a cisternal injection, and it is a time-honored way to treat cocci meningitis. (In his youth, Hans Einstein had been a master of the technique.) A cisternal injection brings amphotericin B directly to the area of maximum meningitis, but it also brings a long spinal needle within millimeters of the upper spinal cord and brain stem. It is a dangerous procedure.

In addition, I started Roger on a new medication taken by mouth called fluconazole. No oral medication had ever had any effect on cocci meningitis, but this new drug looked promising. I didn't want to rely on fluconazole alone, but I hoped Roger would benefit from its added effects.

Now Roger embarked upon the most difficult phase of his treatment. Twice a week his father drove him to the hospital. He had to lie on his stomach in the fluoroscopy suite while the neuro-radiologist injected the base of his brain with amphotericin B. The injections were painful and frightening. I remember him, wet with sweat and tremulous, lying as still as he could on the cold, black table. I was glad that after the first few injections the neuroradiologists didn't need me to be present for the procedure.

These treatments went on for three months, during which time Roger's cocci meningitis improved steadily. Then one Sunday afternoon in February, I was standing in line at a bookstore with my children when my beeper went off. It was one of the doctors on call in the emergency room.

"Are you following a patient named Roger Grove who's getting cisternal injections?"

"Yes," I replied with rising dread.

"His father brought him to the ER this afternoon. He's pretty sick with vomiting and blurry vision, and he's got severe weakness from the waist down. He can't walk. I'm admitting him to the high-acuity ward and getting an MRI of his brain."

I stood there with my cell phone glued to my ear listening to the ER doc go through this dispassionate description of disaster. It was obvious what was going on. Roger, who had been injected the previous day, must have bled into his spinal cord.

Besides the weakness in his legs, Roger had little feeling in his feet and was unable to control his bladder or his bowels. When I arrived at his bedside, a catheter had been inserted to drain his urine. Roger was so scared his voice was shaky but he managed a weak smile.

The neurologist started a cortisone compound in high dose by vein to decrease the inflammatory damage of the blood on the spinal tissue. On the MRI, the neuroradiologist, Dr. Drabkin, showed me the area that might have been damaged during Roger's last cisternal injection. Only a tiny abnormality was visible, but it was in a critical location in the cervical spinal cord. I told Dr. Drabkin, "I know you feel terrible, but this kid didn't have a chance without your help."

Fortunately, Roger began to improve by the next day. First the power started to return to his legs. Then he regained control of his bladder and bowels, and he was able to go home with a walker soon after. With physical therapy, his strength gradually came back.

He regained most of the sensation in his feet, although this took the longest time to recover. His bowels were never quite the same; he had a tendency toward constipation.

I abandoned Roger's cisternal injections. I had lost my nerve. I decided to treat him with high doses of fluconazole alone. I didn't realize it at the time, but fluconazole was turning out to be the big breakthrough treatment for cocci meningitis. Roger was my last patient to have cisternal injections for this disease.

Five years passed and Roger did reasonably well. He came to see me in the office about every three months, and I came to know and like him. Roger had no malice or guile and he was shy, so I knew to keep the personal questions to a minimum. It wasn't until we started discussing his passion, the Civil War, that I realized his intellect. In his free time, he read about the Confederacy, traveled to Civil War sites, and worked out at the gym.

Then one day in 1996 he came to my clinic complaining of a pain inside his abdomen where the shunt tubing ended. His headaches had also returned. After several months of inconclusive tests, it became obvious that Roger's shunt was failing. The system must have become plugged, not an uncommon problem with these shunts because the body reacts to the foreign material and covers it with protein.

Dr. Arian took Roger back to the operating room and replaced his shunt tubing. The evening after the surgery Roger seemed to be doing fine and was able to walk around his room. He was scheduled to go home the next day. But late that night he suddenly became short of breath and collapsed. The doctor on call rushed to his bedside. A lung scan was ordered looking for a blood clot, but none was found. Roger was moved into intensive care. The next morning he was in a coma, and despite our best efforts, he would not wake up. He died a few days later. Dr. Arian believed the most likely cause of death was a rare complication of brain surgery called neurogenic pulmonary edema, where the lungs swell in reaction to disturbing the brain. But for Roger's father, Jack, and for me, it had all happened too suddenly. It was as if Roger had disappeared into thin air.

And so I went to another cocci funeral. After the service in the chapel we went to the graveside on a grassy hill under a tree. Only a few months before, Roger had told his father that if he died, he wanted to be buried in that cemetery. The headstone Jack had made for Roger had two cats on it, one on either side of his name.

Jack gave me some of Roger's Civil War books, which I put in my living room where I can see them every day, because what I do with my deceased patients is remember them. I keep them. I still see Jack occasionally (he has been admitted to the hospital several times with heart disease). The last time I talked to him he asked me if I ever found out exactly what killed Roger. I had to tell him no.

As time went on, it became apparent from our own experience and from published studies that, in most patients, high dose fluconazole alone was effective in controlling cocci meningitis. Very few people these days get injections of amphotericin B into the central nervous system. For me, Roger was a cusp patient—the last to get amphotericin B injections at the base of his brain, the first to get fluconazole only. Today, the most traumatic treatments have largely disappeared, and, except in the very elderly, cocci meningitis has become a manageable disease instead of an inevitable death sentence.

Can cocci meningitis ever be cured? Dr. Daniel Dewsnup and his colleagues, all physicians working with cocci patients in central

California, gathered detailed information on eighteen patients with cocci meningitis who, for one reason or another, were no longer taking fluconazole. In the February 1996 article in the *Annals of Internal Medicine*, they reported that of the eighteen patients, fourteen eventually relapsed with cocci after their treatment was stopped. These relapses occurred as early as two weeks and as late as thirty months after treatment was discontinued; there seemed to be no way to predict which patients were at highest risk. They concluded that the drug doesn't cure, but only suppresses cocci and that "discontinuing azole therapy is unsafe."

Patients get tired of taking their fluconazole, sick of the thin hair and chapped lips it causes, and sometimes they stop the little pink pills, thinking the cocci won't notice. But if the cocci is in the brain, there's almost always a relapse. When my cocci meningitis patients ask me about stopping treatment, I have to tell them that their disease is under control, but it's not gone.

It is late November in Southern California, Thanksgiving week. I take out the trash and walk back across the driveway. The top of our big ash tree tosses violently in the wind. Flying horizontal in the southeast, the constellation Orion is shining brilliantly in a sky blown clear of smog. This is when the cocci spores are carried aloft, and in Simi Valley, or Northridge, or on my own street in Encino, someone, somewhere, is inhaling a lungful of cocci.

chapter 4

a*i*ds

The day I thought I'd contracted HIV was a Thursday in June 1989; I was working at the clinic at the VA hospital. The sun was streaming through the open windows in the big exam room in building ten, and the view was of grass, sycamore trees, and a yard where the nursing home dog barked behind a white picket fence.

Dudley was a tall African-American with advanced AIDS and Kaposi's sarcoma. Flat maroon tumors lay just under his skin like tongues. HIV had burnt out the nerves going down his long legs. When he walked he couldn't feel his feet, and at night, tingling, burning, and shooting pains disturbed his sleep.

He was lying on his back on an examination table. His wild black hair seemed too big for his face and his temples were sunken, but his brown eyes followed my movements with cheerful alertness.

I broke a wooden tongue depressor in half to create a sharp splinter and said, "Dudley, I want to check the sensation in your legs and feet. Tell me if this feels sharp or dull."

I moved down his legs poking the skin between his tumors, but whether I jabbed lightly or with force, all he said was, "Dull, dull, dull."

I do my job out of habit, like most people. So when Dudley couldn't feel my jabs, I wondered if something was wrong with my wooden stick, and forgetting that I was in the AIDS clinic, I absent-mindedly tested it against my own left palm.

The splinter sticking out of the end went right through my skin. I looked with horror as a drop of blood beaded up just milli-meters from a big vein. The stick was as sharp as a needle! If it went through my skin, it had been going into Dudley's HIV-saturated tissues over and over again, only he hadn't been able to feel it.

I excused myself and walked out of the room in a daze. The clinic chief and some ID fellows and residents were standing in the hall. "I stuck myself," I said. They stopped talking and followed me into an empty exam room where I pumped soap on my palm from a dispenser and plunged it under hot water. Someone reached for a bottle of alcohol and poured it over my hand. The wound was in-visible now, but my body's defenses had been breached. Suddenly, my head started to pound and I felt a buffeting in my ears like beating wings. The concerned voices of my colleagues became dim as they led me to a chair and I sat down.

Then I had to tell the clinic chief what I'd done. Looking up at a circle of anxious faces, I had to confess my colossal carelessness. It's not every day that a physician pokes herself with an HIV-contaminated sharp stick almost on purpose.

"It's a low-risk injury, because the stick wasn't visibly bloody," my chief said, "but it's bad enough for you to go on AZT." We were all thinking the same thing. The risk of my getting the infection was less than a half of one percent, but the chance of survival if I was infected was zero.

I wasn't even supposed to be working in the HIV clinic. I was supposed to be running the emergency room and limiting my ID work to a couple of months a year on the inpatient consultation service. But that had been before my friend Henry became ill with AIDS.

Henry was a gay oncologist in Connecticut, and before I got married, he'd been my best friend. We met at Pomona College where we were both pre-med. Henry was tall and thin, with soft blond hair that grew over his collar and a booming laugh you could hear all the way out in the courtyard. He had a wicked sense of humor and spent way too much time playing bridge.

When Henry didn't get into medical school he thought it was the worst thing that could have happened to him. After graduating from Pomona he went to Boston to work in a lab, and I started med school in New Haven. Two times a month I took the train or bummed a ride to visit him. We walked around Concord where he was staying, drank scotch at bars in Boston, and talked about Marcel Proust and Henry James. I didn't know Henry was gay, and I don't think he was clear on that point yet, either. Homosexuality was a dim concept to me then. I was just trying to figure out why we weren't sleeping together.

Henry finally came out in 1975, and by that time, he was a medical student at the University of Southern California. The next year I came back to Los Angeles to do my residency, and on the weekends we went to the bars in West Hollywood. In the frenzy of gay liberation and discomania, we joined the lines of dancers at Oil

Can Harry's or at Studio One. It took Henry a couple of years to find Mike, a businessman who'd been a diabetic since childhood. They were a good match—politically conservative sons of well-to-do families, they had the same values.

Henry and Mike got along well with Glenn, my college boyfriend who became my husband, and after they moved to the East Coast, they made it a point to come out for a visit once or twice a year. I have a picture of Henry holding my infant son, Paul, slightly away from his body, with an uncomfortable smile as if he didn't have confidence in Paul's diaper.

I don't remember the first time I made the connection between Henry and the new patients we were starting to see on the wards—people with a lung disease that wasn't supposed to occur in normal adults. All of the ID docs read the article in the *New England Journal of Medicine* that appeared in the December 10 issue in 1981, a report by Michael Gottlieb that described five gay males, all of whom had been admitted to the UCLA Medical Center with the same strange pneumonia—*Pneumocystis carinii* pneumonia, or PCP for short. PCP had killed malnourished infants in European orphanages after World War II, and we occasionally saw it in cancer patients after chemo, but not in seemingly healthy adults from the community. These new patients had PCP in every part of their lungs.

On closer questioning, they told their doctors they'd had weight loss and diarrhea for months before their PCP. Soon, similar patients began turning up in New York and San Francisco. The numbers were small; I was more intrigued at first than concerned.

But by 1982, a steady stream of patients with PCP were coming into the emergency room. All of them were either gay men, IV drug abusers, or their girlfriends. It was the quiet beginning of an epidemic.

I had a new job then teaching interns and residents at the Sepulveda Veterans Hospital and at the Olive View County Hospital. My residents and I made rounds on one young man in the intensive care unit at Olive View. David was a musician, about twenty-four years old, with wavy brown hair and blue eyes. He wasn't gay, and his concerned girlfriend was with him all the time, but he had used intravenous drugs.

Within twenty-four hours Dave was gasping for breath on a 100-percent oxygen mask, but he had confidence in me. Just before my residents put in the endotracheal tube and attached him to the ventilator machine, he said, "I know you're going to pull me through, Doc." He thought he was too young to die, but he was wrong. His lungs were too clogged and damaged by Pneumocystis to let him take in any oxygen. Like many of these new PCP arrivals, he lasted only a few days on the ventilator before he succumbed to his infection.

The new disease was called the acquired immune deficiency syndrome because the collapse in the patients' immune systems seemed to be caused by some factor the patients acquired in adult life, but what this factor was remained a complete mystery. All the patients had abnormally low numbers of a type of white blood cell, the helper T lymphocyte. People normally have at least one thousand of these cells in every milliliter of blood. AIDS patients with PCP usually had less than two hundred. These T lymphocytes seemed to be important in the defense against certain kinds of infections. Not only did persons with AIDS have PCP; they had genital

herpes outbreaks that didn't heal. The little blisters became excruci-
ating, painful, deep ulcers, with extensive loss of tissue. And AIDS
patients proved very susceptible to tuberculosis, which multiplied in
their bodies at a rapid rate and quickly spread beyond the confines
of the lungs. *Candida albicans,* the cause of minor vaginal yeast infections, formed extensive and uncomfortable white patches in their
throats. Exotic fungi like *Cryptococcus,* once rare, invaded their brains.

Beyond infections, individuals with AIDS came down with
strange cancers, like Dudley's Kaposi's sarcoma. Up until this point,
Kaposi's sarcoma had been a rare tumor that appeared on the legs
of old men. In AIDS patients it involved the entire body inside and
out. These patients also succumbed to aggressive tumors of the
blood cells, like lymphomas. All of these infections and malignan-
cies could be traced to one problem: the T helper cell, an important
line of defense, was being destroyed by something in the blood of
our AIDS patients.

Researchers advanced all sorts of theories about what caused
the disease. One such theory blamed amyl nitrate "poppers," small
capsules that when popped and inhaled release a whiff of pungent
gas that stimulates the heart, and is thought by many in the gay
community to enhance orgasm. But such ideas fell by the wayside as
first the drug users, then other non-gay patients appeared: heterosexual Haitians, patients with hemophilia who received blood products, patients who had received transfusions, and the heterosexual
partners of infected persons. Most scientists believed that the cause
of AIDS was some kind of infectious agent, transmitted by blood
and by body fluids. But none of the methods used to isolate bacteria
and viruses were successful in finding the cause of the infection.

One of the satisfactions of working in infectious diseases had been the sure knowledge that with cool heads and a fund of information, we could diagnose difficult cases and then offer a cure. In what other specialty could the doctor say to the patient: I'll clear up this infection and in a week you'll be as good as new. But AIDS was a blow to the heart, a mystery wrapped in fear for which we had little to offer.

We became expert at treating all the bizarre infections these patients came down with, like a parasite from cats called toxoplasmosis that destroyed the brain from the inside. We fought off a virus infection of the retina called cytomegalovirus or CMV that caused blindness. People commonly carry CMV all their lives without any symptoms, but AIDS allows the virus to multiply out of control. Many patients went through illness after illness, returning to the clinic after each bout, thinner and weaker than before. One man developed massive swelling in his legs because HIV had weakened his heart muscle, causing fluid to back up in his limbs. He was in his late twenties, but he looked much older. They all looked like they had aged prematurely.

Month in and month out, we waited with our patients. We found out how courageous they could be, gay and straight. They were afraid, and they were also objects of fear. But I learned that there was a limit to how sad or frightened patients could get. They mostly adapted and went on one day at a time.

One man, who was like a character out of a Damon Runyon story, said, "I got AIDS from hookers." When I met Bobby, his T cell count was about 250, so with good treatment, he had some years of life left. But HIV had damaged the long nerves in his right leg. Although he felt well in every other respect, he was never without pain. Despite this he was a tough little guy, always cheerful and upbeat. "I'm alive and kicking," he'd say, leaning against his cane.

Eventually, we got better at preventing infections in patients whose T cells had been consumed by a fire we were helpless to put out. But the end was always the same. We felt more like oncologists than ID doctors, writing triplicate prescriptions for narcotics for intractable pain and schooling ourselves in end-of-life issues like hospice care.

Our own fear was hard to control. While AIDS did not appear to be contagious by casual contact, in the early days no one was certain. I was reluctant to greet patients by shaking hands. Routine events became terrifying. One afternoon, before my adventure with Dudley, I was with my residents making rounds at the bedside of a patient in the terminal stage of AIDS. In his delirium, he grabbed the plastic tubing from the bag of antibiotic that was plugged into his intravenous line and wrapped it around his fingers. There was a long needle at the end that was used to make the connection into his IV. Alarmed that the patient might injure himself, I began to extricate the intravenous tubing and needle from his hands. The patient made a sudden movement. The needle flew up and I felt its sharp touch along my palm like lightning. I was lucky that time; there was no break in the skin. But it was a terrifying experience.

At first we'd seen only people in the late stages of the disease, but over time we began to see gay men with swollen lymph glands and mild fever. And although there was no blood test yet, we suspected that they, too, were infected with the unknown agent. One of my young interns, a gay man, took me aside one day in clinic.

"I've got these swollen lymph nodes, boss," he said with a sad smile.

It was a long two years before French and American investigators isolated the human immunodeficiency virus, the cause of AIDS, in 1984, and another year until the first drug—zidovudine, or AZT—was developed to attack the millions of copies of the virus that are present in white blood cells of infected patients. In that interminable, terrible time, like everyone with gay friends, I often prayed that no one I knew, especially Henry, would develop even a cold. But it seemed it was impossible to avoid being touched by the disease. The obituary pages filled with the names of the young.

As we learned more about the disease, it became clear to me that AIDS had been moving silently among us when I was spending time with Henry in the gay community in the 1970s. The patients who had first shown up at UCLA in 1980 had been slowly burning with the disease for at least two years and probably more than four.

But it took me a long time to realize, and perhaps admit, that Henry was sick. In the mid-1980s he developed arthritis in his back and knees. I worried that it was HIV-related, but I didn't bring it up. I didn't want to face the possibility. Then around 1987, Henry's personality changed. He became quiet; he didn't do that sudden whirl of his, leaning over and grinning when he told stories. He stood still when he talked, and his laugh disappeared.

One fall morning in 1988, he called me from Connecticut. "Pam, I've got a fever," he said, "and I don't think I'm breathing right." Actually, he was so short of breath he couldn't complete a sentence.

"Henry, have you had an HIV test? I think you have Pneumo-cystis pneumonia." He hadn't been tested. He was living a secret life in his small community.

"I want you to treat me," he said.

"You mean, over the phone?"

"Yes," he answered.

"You've got to go see a doctor."

"I can't," he said. "Not in my town. No one knows I'm gay. I have patients. They won't understand."

I told Henry what pills to take. He was sick enough to be in the hospital but somehow he pulled through.

A few weeks later, I rearranged my schedule in the emergency room so I could attend the HIV clinic every Thursday morning. Maybe I'd been holding back before, not wanting to get my hands dirty. A lot of ID doctors were reluctant to get involved with HIV in those days, and some of them never did. They split HIV off from their specialty and set up separate clinics, run by gay male MDs with an interest in the disease. But not at the VA. The ID department had jumped right in, and I was ready to join them.

It wasn't just Henry's illness that drew me into the fray. I knew I was part of the biggest infectious disease emergency since the in-fluenza pandemic of 1918. I'd been reading a biography of Isak Dinesen, the Danish woman who wrote *Out of Africa*. She took as her motto the two words in Renaissance French on her lover's family crest, *"Je responderai."* And that's how it was for me. I could hear a battle going on and cries for help, and I remember thinking, "I will answer."

It had been some sixty minutes since my accident. I was standing at the drinking fountain next to the pharmacy window swallowing my first two blue-and-white AZT capsules. I'd be taking two capsules every four hours around the clock for the next six weeks to try and prevent any HIV carried into my body attaching to my cells and starting the fatal cycle of infection.

As I finished my morning clinic I hurried home to take four-year-old Paul to nursery school. I walked through my front door, dropping down on one knee to nuzzle him and his two-year-old sister, realizing that if I got AIDS, I'd be leaving them in their early teens.

During the first week on the drug, I was intensely anxious and preoccupied. It didn't help that I had to take medicine every four hours around the clock. It was when the alarm went off at 3 A.M. that I realized my problem had me on a very short leash.

But I'm convinced that human beings can adapt to anything. About four days after the accident, I was pumping gas, and as I stood gazing off into space, I realized that I wasn't thinking about anything. My problem was now a faint whispering I could hear in the background, but the rest of my mind was free to think about anything or nothing.

I had at least six weeks to wait, the usual incubation period following an exposure like mine to HIV. If infection did set in, there might be sore throat, fever, rash, and body aches. All I felt was some nausea, and a little buzz in my head from the drug.

Every two weeks, I reported to the lab for a complete blood count to make sure I was tolerating the medicine. After four weeks of therapy, I sat down at the computer in the ER to check the results from that morning's test. As I scrolled through the green numbers, one jumped out. Circulating white blood cells called the polymorphonu-clear leukocytes, or polys for short, are essential for life. They func-tion like kamikaze pilots, jumping on germs, immolating them and dying in the process. But AZT, like chemotherapy, can drop the poly count from the normal 6,000 to below 500, where serious infection is almost inevitable. I realized with a start that I had only 700 polys! Another day or two on the drug and I'd have been a sitting duck for infection. So I stopped the AZT and waited out the rest of my time.

I was working in the ER a month later when the lab supervi-sor called me with the final test result. "Pam, your HIV antibody is negative." Five minutes later my heart was still pounding, but I knew I was in the clear.

When I started my new job at the HMO, Henry was in the final stages of his disease. He had seizures and he was losing his vi-sion to CMV. During his last visit to California, he lay on my living room floor with his head on a pillow listening to Glenn, Mike, and me talk. My mother gave him some chicken soup, and he leaned on one elbow to spoon some of it in his mouth and then sank back again too tired to eat. He died a few months later. The last time I talked to him on the phone I was in a hurry to get my kids to school. "I'll talk to you tomorrow," I said. He seemed reluctant to hang up. I'm still haunted by that conversation because he knew it would be our last but I didn't.

It was 1989, and my patients and I had seven more years to en-dure without real hope. The available drugs were too similar to be active against HIV for more than a year or so. Viruses reproducing rapidly inside the cells of the host accumulate tiny changes in their RNA and eventually the viruses produced are resistant to the drugs.

So many people died, waiting for the medicines that would finally help them.

One day the paramedics brought in a patient of mine with advanced AIDS to the hospital. Kaposi's sarcoma tumors had invaded Jim's lungs, and he could no longer breathe. His face was distorted and purple with the same tumors. The ER doctor intubated him and put him on a ventilator. Although Jim couldn't talk because of the tube in his throat, he was able to tell me by writing on a tablet that he understood his condition was hopeless and he wanted to die. We arranged for his family to come in the early afternoon. I told him I would return to the ICU and take the tube out of his throat when I finished my morning clinic.

Jim had been a friend of another gay man, Jerry, who used to cut my hair for years. He was a lanky fellow who really wanted to be a chiropractor, and who liked to practice manipulations on my sore neck. When I moved to the San Fernando Valley, I lost track of him. Then Jim told me Jerry had died of AIDS.

I don't know if I believe in an afterlife or not, but at that moment, I really thought Jim would pass on into the next world. As I prepared to take his tube out, I said to Jim, "When you get to the other side, say 'Hello' to Jerry from me."

I held Jim's hand and asked him if he was ready. He smiled and signaled that he was. His lover and his family were standing around the bed.

Then I said, "Goodbye," and took the tube out while the respiratory therapist suctioned his airway clear of secretions. Now it was time for me to go. Reluctantly and with a tight chest, I left him with his family and closed the door behind me.

Finally, at the end of 1995 the first new class of anti-HIV drugs was released—the protease inhibitors. They inhibited replication of HIV in a powerful new way, and when combined with the older drugs it took much longer for the virus to develop resistance to their effects. The new drug regimens brought some very sick patients back, almost from the brink of death. One woman, who had contracted HIV from a blood transfusion she received when her daughter was born, had CMV retinitis, cryptococcal meningitis, and a chronic infection of the blood stream that had enlarged her liver and spleen and made her dependent on regular blood transfusions. All of these infections went into remission on the new drugs. Her liver and spleen returned to their normal size; she gained weight and went back to work.

The patients who come to see me now are often long-term survivors whose present appearance gives little clue to the muscle wasting, the terrifying pneumonias, and devouring herpes infections they suffered before we had strong drug combinations. I met one patient after she was intubated and put on a ventilator for PCP. Now she has regained all the weight she lost and is taking care of her three children.

Another patient, who was once covered with purple Kaposi's tumors, works for a few months each year and then hits the road in a Mustang convertible. "I'm a shameless extrovert," he says, his bright round face beaming with pleasure. He almost lost his life once, and he refuses to be a slave to his job or to have a gloomy attitude. He's learned what healthy people often never realize, that life is a party and he is the guest of honor.

Another patient of mine is a husky fellow with intense blue eyes and a short brown beard, like a sailor. The new drugs brought him back from a T cell count of fewer than fifty. He and his HIV-negative partner practice safe sex and are the responsible parents of two boys, adopted from Russia as infants.

"Are they twins?" I ask.

"They are now," he answers.

He painted a beautiful picture in silver and blue that hangs in one of my examination rooms and has a line from the movie *The In-Laws*. Peter Falk, playing an FBI agent, is trying to recruit a soda jerk into the agency while being shot at by the bad guys through the store window. He's going on about the pension plan and the dental plan but then he has to add that, "Survival is the key to the benefits program."

In the early days of the new drugs, the atmosphere in the HIV clinic was like a party. Life came back. We all wanted to believe the worst was over, and that it wouldn't be returning. But we're beginning to see the limits of the miracle, the difficulty of sustaining it.

Not long ago our clinic coordinator received a distraught phone call from one of my patients, Carey, a diabetic with HIV. His partner, Alan, had walked to the warehouse store about a mile from their apartment and on his way home he had gotten lost and wandered around for hours. Carey called the police. Late that night Alan came through the door: hungry, tired, and confused. Alan had been off HIV therapy for about a year. He had become tired of drug side effects and he felt better off treatment. But his count of virus particles, the viral load, had climbed inexorably and he had been losing weight. When Carey brought Alan into clinic the week after he had gotten lost, it was obvious he was suffering from AIDS dementia complex. This is an insidious process in which HIV invades the brain and sabotages all of its programs: reasoning, emotion, and personality. Alan, who is a brilliant freelance computer programmer, sat on my examination table wasted, with sunken temples. He answered my questions with sparse half-sentences, his features an immobile mask. Even his ability to feel fear about the direction his illness was taking was dulled by the virus multiplying inside his brain. But his partner was distraught.

The HIV pharmacist and I started three drugs with good penetration in the brain. Five weeks later the two men returned to clinic for their appointments. Alan had gained fifteen pounds, his temples had filled out, and his eyes were alive again. He was like a person who had been released from some evil enchantment. Carey, sitting on the exam table for his appointment, thanked us for what we'd been able to do.

"We had a friend staying with us last week," Carey said, "and I asked him to wake me early one morning in case I overslept. He said, 'OK, but Alan is very protective of your sleep, you know.' And that really touched me. I felt like going in and hugging Alan because I knew he really cared about me. It was terrible when he was so lost, and it's wonderful to have him back."

I remembered my friend Henry and his lover then, and how Henry had told me about a year after he met Mike, "He couldn't like me better." I wished we could have done something when the HIV attacked Henry's wonderful mind. He suffered secretly for years, but he must have taken some precautions, because he never infected Mike, who, sadly, died of diabetic complications a few years after him. Nowadays we could have done more for Henry, and maybe he wouldn't have been afraid to ask for help.

None of the new drugs, including the newest ones, the non-nucleoside reverse transcriptase inhibitors, are a cure for HIV disease. The virus is always present in some cells of the body, and if the patients stop taking all of their drugs, as Alan did, or even worse, skip some doses of some of the drugs in their cocktail, it begins to reproduce again, often in a resistant and hard-to-treat form. And even the most conscientious patients, who swallow handfuls of pills at exactly the right time, will eventually develop a resistant strain of HIV in their bodies, which through natural selection will become the predominant one.

— It's humbling to know how short the reach of even this treatment has been. By the end of 1999 there were an estimated thirty-three million adults and children in the world living with HIV, 90 percent of them in the developing world, and 70 percent of those in Africa. AIDS has caused about sixteen million deaths, and every day there are approximately sixteen thousand new infections. In poor countries, HIV is transmitted by heterosexual contact and by intravenous drug use. Infection rates are rising rapidly in girls and young women who are infected by older men. Worldwide, AIDS has created nine million orphaned children. Drug companies are only beginning to make available discounted or donated medicines to control transmission of HIV from mother to child and antibiotics to prevent infections like tuberculosis and cryptococcal meningitis in HIV-infected Africans.

Until there is a vaccine that eliminates HIV transmission the way the smallpox vaccine wiped out smallpox, AIDS, like syphilis,

will always be a "shadow on the land." Even a drug that could eliminate every HIV particle from the body of an infected person wouldn't
be enough, because sexually transmitted diseases can never be elimi-
nated by medical treatment alone. A steady stream of new cases always
keeps such diseases alive. Despite hundreds of years of indoctrina-
tion about the dangers of venereal diseases, far too many people do
not take the necessary precautions.

And so the infections, and the deaths, continue. My HIV
clinic meets two half-days a week and the flow of cases never
ceases. Along with my boss, Dr. Debra Sachs, and our clinic nurses,
the treatment team includes our HIV coordinator, a pharmacist, a
dietitian, and a social worker—HIV treatment has become too
complex for me to manage alone. But that hasn't changed the way I
feel when I meet a new patient in clinic for the first time. From the
minute we shake hands—I'm not afraid to do that now—I know
that we're beginning a long relationship that's going to get closer as
the disease progresses. In some cases, I'm going to be with the patient until the last day of his or her life.

About twice a year I get my AIDS dream. I don't think it will
ever go away. In my dream I realize that my negative blood test was
a mistake, that all the time I have really been getting sicker and
sicker without knowing it. I become thin and develop a strange
cancer, and I realize I'm going to die soon of AIDS. I gather my
children around me, because I have to tell them what I have. Then
I wake up, but the doomed feeling hangs over me for hours.

Since I've been a doctor I've lost many patients, but always just
a small number to any one disease. With AIDS it's different. Like
Ulysses when he visited the underworld, my memories throng me.

I can see Jim in the ICU saying goodbye to his family, and my young intern with the swollen glands smiling through his fear. I remember Bobby limping on his sore leg with his cane in his right hand and one of those cakes he used to bring in his left. And then there's Henry and me walking down Charles Street on a spring afternoon. It's still cool enough for him to wear his soft wool topcoat. I grab his arm and pull him into a bookstore, and we're happy because we're going to have a nice supper later and because we're going to be friends forever.

maneater

In 1989 the Rocky Mountain Pus Club, a group of infectious disease specialists headed by Dennis Stevens in Boise, Idaho, published an article in the *New England Journal of Medicine* that described severe streptococcal infections in twenty patients living in Montana, Idaho, Utah, and Nevada. The patients Stevens described were in their mid-thirties. Thirteen of them had been in good health, two consumed "liberal amounts of alcohol," one had diabetes mellitus, and the others had miscellaneous medical conditions.

All of them had suddenly become ill, with severe pain, usually in an arm or leg, accompanied by fever, chills, body aches, and sometimes vomiting and diarrhea. They went into shock quickly, often within four hours of being admitted to the hospital, and they deteriorated fast. Their kidneys failed, they became confused, and their lungs filled with fluid. If they survived, most of them went to the operating room so doctors could take a closer look at their infected limbs, which were swollen, red, and in some cases, covered with large blisters filled with serum and blood.

When the surgeons cut open these areas, they found that the group A strep bacterium—the same one that's responsible for sore throats—had invaded the tough connective tissue known as the fascia, which penetrates and supports the muscles from below the skin down to the bone. The tissue was dead, and the bacteria and the dying fascia were releasing toxins that were killing the patient. Antibiotics alone could not stop this process. If the patient were to survive, the surgeons had to remove all involved tissue, whether it was an arm, a leg, or even part of the abdominal wall. Thirty percent of the patients died, despite maximum surgical and medical treatment.

What had killed their tissues, and them, was necrotizing fasciitis: "flesh-eating strep."

"Flesh-eating strep" sounds like something that belongs on the pages of *Weekly World News* along with the aliens and Elvis sightings, but it's actually one of the ferociously lethal strains of an old human nemesis. And unlike those Elvis sightings, it's all too real.

Group A strep, or *Streptococcus pyogenes*, is one of humankind's ancient enemies. When people used to talk about "blood poisoning" from a wound, the usual culprit was the group A strep. It was one of the causes of gangrene that followed amputations during the Civil War, and a leading cause of death after surgery in the 1800s, when anesthesia made long operations possible, but lack of sterility made the patients easy targets for bacteria. On the surgical wards they called what killed post-op patients "hospitalism," but it was mostly infection by group A strep, and it killed nurses and doctors as well.

Strep was responsible for childbed fever, an invasive infection of the pelvic organs and blood stream that took the lives of new mothers for centuries, and for scarlet fever, a complication of strep throat that caused severe illness and sometimes death in children.

After sulfa drugs were introduced in the late 1930s, and penicillin a decade later, the death rate from serious group A strep infections plummeted. These terrors of our grandparents: septic scarlet fever, childbed fever, and streptococcal gangrene became rare. Rheumatic fever, a form of heart disease that follows strep throat, almost disappeared in the developed world.

Then in the mid-1980s doctors around the world began to report fatal strep cases. Dr. Stevens's report came out in 1989, and the next year, Muppet-creator Jim Henson died of group A strep pneumonia, a disease that was rarely seen in adults. Henson, fifty-three, had been fighting a "cold" through the weekend. He told his daughter, Lisa, he was just tired, but by Monday evening he was coughing up blood. That night he was admitted to New York Hospital in Manhattan. Despite treatment with multiple antibiotics, his lungs, kidneys, heart, and blood-clotting systems all failed, and in less than twenty-four hours he was dead.

Reports followed from Kansas in 1991, and Sweden and Ontario, Canada, in 1992. Then in 1994 invasive group A strep infections came to public attention when an outbreak in Gloucestershire, England, killed at least seven and as many as ten people. The British tabloids published lurid accounts of the victims' sufferings and dubbed the syndrome "flesh-eating strep."

Particularly disturbing was that the illness started with the most trivial injuries, the kind all of us experience in our everyday lives. One patient was scratched on the arm by her dog; another sustained a paper cut. That was all it took for this bacterium, whose normal home is the human throat and skin, to get into the patients' bodies and to invade the deeper tissues. Occasional cases were traced to insect bites, but in these patients the insect was not the strep carrier; it just made the tiny hole through which the germ got in.

Anxious patients began to ask their doctors how they could protect themselves from group A strep infections. The problem couldn't be attacked with a mop and disinfectant because this germ does not survive long in an inanimate environment. People don't catch "flesh-eating step" from dust, clothing, or blankets. Transmission by food or water is also rare.

Group A strep is spread from one person to another (with an occasional case traced to the family dog), and the most efficient transmitter is a child who is carrying it in his throat. Children with acute strep throat discharge tiny droplets of saliva and nasal secretions loaded with the germ into the air, and these are inhaled by the adults and children around them. They in turn become temporary carriers and infect others, both in the throat and on the skin. On average, from 15 to 20 percent of normal school children are carrying group A strep in their throats at any given time, and many never develop symptoms. So, in counseling patients and their families, doctors can only recommend avoiding close contact with children with sore throats and carefully washing cuts and scrapes and covering them with a clean bandage. There is, however, no sure way to avoid getting group A strep.

Fortunately, you're more likely to get strep throat from someone else than "flesh-eating strep." Nevertheless, person-to-person transmission of this infection does occasionally occur. On June 11, 1994, a forty-six-year-old woman was admitted to Akron General Hospital in Ohio with severe pain in her right elbow. She did not mention any injury to her arm; however, since she was already going into shock at the time of her admission, she may have been unable to describe the details of her illness. Her blood pressure was low (a state of septic shock), and she was covered from head to toe with a scarlet fever rash. The area surrounding her right elbow was red, swollen, and very tender. This patient recovered with just antibiotics and drainage of the fluid around her elbow, but her seventy-three-year-old father-in-law was not so lucky.

On June 28 he came to the clinic with severe pain in his right hand. There was no redness and no swelling so the physician on duty diagnosed a torn ligament and sent him home with a splint and pain medication. Two days later the patient returned in shock. His right hand was swollen and covered with large blisters. While the physicians in the emergency room watched in horror, the skin of his arm turned maroon all the way to his shoulder. Three hours later he was in the operating room having his arm amputated. His right flank then turned maroon and the tissue died through the muscle to the abdominal wall. Cultures of his blood and tissues were just turning positive for group A strep when, forty-eight hours after they were drawn, the patient died.

Other instances of person-to-person spread of "flesh-eating strep" within families have also been reported, and a fascinating case of transmission from a patient to a health care worker was reported in the *Annals of Emergency Medicine*. In 1990, firemen were called to the home of a three-year-old boy in cardiopulmonary arrest. One firefighter used a handheld mask to propel oxygen-rich air into the lungs of the child. Despite their best efforts the boy died en route to the emergency room. During the resuscitation, the fireman's "hands were covered with the patient's sputum, and when subsequently cleaning his equipment, he struck the dorsum of his right hand against a wall, resulting in a small abrasion."

The following day the fireman was vomiting and had chills and a fever. By the time his wife brought him in the next day he was covered with a red rash and was in early shock. There was a hard red wound on his right hand with darker red streaks going up his arm. Fortunately, this fireman recovered after a week in the hospital, and he got to keep his arm. Both his wound and the tissues of the fatally infected three-year-old grew group A strep.

The three streptococcal syndromes—necrotizing fasciitis, childbed fever, and scarlet fever—are all caused by a family of toxins the bacteria manufacture in the human body. But group A strep can cause two other diseases indirectly. In rheumatic fever, antibodies manufactured by the body against group A strep turn instead against the heart, joints, and brain. In Bright's disease, other antibodies against the strep attack the patient's kidneys. In both of these syndromes, the heart and kidney damage may be irreversible and eventually fatal. In the developed world, penicillin and newer antibiotics had kept group A strep under control since the 1940s, but in recent years, more virulent new forms have become more common.

It is important to emphasize that not all group A strep infections are life-threatening. Group A strep is still the most common cause of superficial infections of the skin that resolve without treatment or respond promptly to a course of antibiotics by mouth. But the strains of group A strep that cause these mild infections differ from the really virulent strains. Studies of the streptococci isolated from very ill patients like the ones described by Dr. Stevens and his colleagues suggested that group A strep *is* changing. Why this process is happening is unknown. From an evolutionary standpoint, it makes no sense for a parasite to change in a way that results in the rapid death of its host. But in certain lethal strains of group A strep, that is what appears to be happening. These new strep are often rich in M protein, a mucus-like substance in the cell membrane that makes them resistant to being eaten by white blood cells. And some of these strep produced a more powerful form of scarlet fever toxin, similar to the toxins that had caused severe attacks of scarlet fever before 1940. One toxin, pyrogenic exotoxin, not only causes the rash and fever of scarlet fever, but also functions as a superantigen, activating the patient's immune system in disastrous ways. Once activated, hormones are released by the patient's own body that cause kidney function to drop and blood vessels to dilate, plunging the patient into shock, activating the clotting system, and causing both abnormal clots and uncontrolled bleeding.

For me, the case reports on the new killer strep came to life in the spring of 1990, when I was one of three specialists in infectious diseases at my HMO. My friend and colleague, Daniel Lerner, and the section chief, Debra Sachs, were the other specialists. Danny was a balding, chunky man in his late fifties, quiet, even a little shy, and so self-effacing that neither he nor other people always realized how astute he was. But it didn't take me long to figure out that Danny was really good at this special kind of work we do.

On a Saturday in March, the admitting physician asked Danny to see a thirty-six-year-old lawyer named Allan Roth, who was coming to the intensive care unit in the early stages of shock. The admitting physician noted that the patient had a fine red rash that turned pale when pressed. In the right thigh near the groin were two areas of skin that were turning black. The rest of the right groin and upper thigh was hard, red, and tender.

Allan, a tall, athletic lawyer with curly black hair, told the doctors that about seven days before coming into the hospital, he noticed a small insect bite on his right foot, which was probably where the strep entered his body. "I also started to have pain in my right thigh and groin. I thought it was from a hard workout at the gym." He began having nausea, was vomiting, and had body aches, as if he had the flu. "At first I thought I'd get better with rest, but when my thigh became hard and dark red, I knew I had to come in." It was not until the surgeon, Dr. Steven Stein, finished his consultation, that Allan understood how gravely ill he was. He remembers the doctor telling him that he had a very serious infection, remembers him saying, "You may not survive."

Dr. Lerner examined Allan in the intensive care unit. Though he was a calm and experienced senior clinician, not prone to exaggeration, Allan Roth's case filled him with dread and excitement. Allan was not making any urine at all, and his blood tests confirmed that his kidneys were shutting down. So distinctive were the red rash and the darkened skin that, even without culture results, he wrote confidently in the chart: "Severe streptococcal group A disease with pyrogenic exotoxin A and necrotizing fasciitis."

The next Monday he described the case to me, "This guy is really sick, Pam. He's got strep fasciitis, I'm sure of it." He related how the surgeons had rushed Allan to the operating room and removed the whole front of his thigh down to the muscle and the big blood vessels. Dr. Stein cut out all tissue that did not briskly bleed.

Allan Roth did indeed have "flesh-eating strep." Besides causing local damage, the strep bacteria were manufacturing toxins, called pyrogenic exotoxins, that were flooding his blood stream and poisoning his lungs and his kidneys. In the skin over his entire body, the toxins caused a scarlet fever rash, like sunburn roughed up by sandpaper. In the skin and muscles of his infected thigh, group A strep was releasing toxic enzymes that were liquefying everything in their path, clearing the way for bacterial invasion. Group A strep respects no boundaries. If it is not contained, it invades and spreads through tissues, penetrates and dissolves defending lymph nodes, breaks into the blood stream, and along this highway spreads throughout the entire body.

The next morning, Dr. Lerner returned to the intensive care unit to make his rounds. He found Allan alert after his surgery, but still connected to the ventilator. A family of tubes emerged from his body. Working with Danny was a nephrologist who was managing the amounts and types of fluids that were going through all of Allan's intravenous catheters. They both knew that Allan would need immediate kidney dialysis. Not only were his kidneys not functioning, but the strep was causing rapid breakdown of tissue throughout his body. Under infectious attack, Allan's own body was consuming itself. All of these toxins and waste products of metabolism had to be removed if Allan was to recover. The kidney specialist inserted a large plastic catheter into one of the big veins near the collarbone to attach Allan to the kidney machine.

At the bedside was the pulmonary specialist, David Draper. Unusual among doctors, he writes completely legible chart entries. On the day following Allan's surgery, he noted that the patient was "responding appropriately" to questions by gestures. (He could not talk due to the ventilator tube.) The "diffuse erythematous rash" was still present, along with signs of "multisystem failure." Still, since Allan was breathing on his own, Dr. Draper wrote, "will proceed with extubation."

Removing the ventilator tube had a positive effect on Allan's morale. He remembers thinking at the time, "I'm going to make it, I'm not going to die after all."

On the next day, March 19, Dr. Steven Stein took Allan back to the operating room for a second look at his wound. In "flesh-eating strep" this is a customary practice to make sure that no dead tissue remains deep in the infected area. The second debridement, or clean-up surgery, was relatively minor compared with the first. Clearly visible on smears made from the tissue removed at surgery were the blue-staining chains and clumps of group A strep. Strep grew out of Allan's blood cultures as well.

Allan spent over six weeks in the hospital. He required kidney dialysis treatments for most of that time. His wife and three-year-old daughter visited him twice a day. "My daughter seemed to accept my tubes and bandages matter-of-factly," he remembers, "but my six-year-old son was too shaken up by the sight to visit me."

Allan's enormous wound and the processes of tissue break-down and repair required a daily intake of thousands of calories. His wound leaked nutrients even as his body needed high levels of them for manufacturing new tissue to replace what had been destroyed by the group A strep infection. Liquid nutrition, delivered into a large vein in Allan's chest, supplemented his oral feedings. John Teague, the nephrologist, had to carefully manage all of these supplemental fluids to make sure that the dialysis treatments removed just the right amount of fluid from Allan's body.

On March 20, Dr. Draper wrote in the chart that Allan's rash was starting to "desquamate."

"All of my skin peeled off," Allan told me later, "even my tongue!"

During the height of his illness, the scarlet fever toxin had killed the outer layer of Allan's skin. Now he was shedding it like a snake as the new skin pushed the old off his body. But Allan still had a big area of skin and tissue missing from his right thigh and lower abdomen. The muscles were open to the air and were weeping large amounts of serum. Allan was leaking fluids and nutrients; this defect had to be covered. On March 26, a plastic surgeon, Dr. Michael Luskin, joined the team of physicians taking care of Allan.

In his note, he wrote that the patient would need a skin graft, but that the surface of the wound was not ready to take one yet. Cells called granulation tissue migrate onto the surface of large wounds like Allan's. These are the cells that must grab and grow into a skin graft for it to take. Dr. Luskin noted "early granulation only." He added that when there was enough granulation tissue for the wound to appear "beefy," he could cover it with a skin graft.

On April 3, Dr. Luskin went down to the whirlpool bath to examine Allan's wound with the bandages off. Dr. Luskin is a man in his fifties with a neat, gray beard and the clipped accent of his native South Africa. A little forceps always straddles the front pocket of his white coat, and he retains an academic air from his many years as a professor of surgery. Dr. Luskin wrote that the wound was "granulating well." Finally on April 19, one month after he came to the hospital, Allan went back to the operating room where Dr. Luskin covered his terrible wound with a skin graft taken from his left thigh. At first all went well. Then on the third post-operative day, Allan began to have a fever. Cultures of the grafted tissue confirmed what Dr. Luskin already recognized by the telltale fruity odor and blue-green appearance of the pus in the wound.

"Most of graft melted by Pseudomonas," he wrote in the chart.

Pseudomonas aeruginosa, the bacterial enemy of patients with open wounds, had invaded Allan's newly planted graft and was devouring the thin layer of skin cells. Dr. Lerner quickly adjusted Allan's antibiotics. Dr. Luskin ordered irrigation of the area several times a day with special solutions. For Allan, this was a very trying time. "I had a fever every day," he recalls.

Fortunately, by April 26, Allan was doing better. Though most of the skin graft was destroyed, islands of grafted skin did survive the Pseudomonas infection. The nurses began to teach Allan and his wife how to perform the complex dressing changes that he would need at home. Dr. Luskin wrote that Allan could walk with help, and Dr. Lerner noted the fevers were resolving.

Allan still had one major worry: Would his kidneys recover, or would he require permanent dialysis? "Every day I waited for the kidney blood test, the creatinine, to come back. For three weeks I was in suspense." Slowly the creatinine started to fall. Allan's kidneys were recovering.

On May 2, Dr. Lerner stopped Allan's antibiotics, and the next day he went home to continue his convalescence. The healing process took months, but the surviving cells of his graft eventually covered the big wound with a kind of scarred skin. He had to have one more surgery to repair a large hernia that had developed in his weakened abdominal wall, but when that was over, he was able to return to work in his law office. Today a casual observer of his scars would probably guess that he had been the victim of an attack by a large animal, like a shark.

In the years that followed Allan Roth's case of "flesh-eating strep," I had my own cases with group A strep. My patients did not have long hospital stays like Allan. They crashed and burned quickly. The first patient had group A strep pneumonia, like Jim Henson. The patient, a forty-one-year-old man, had only been in the hospital for two days when I was called, but his lungs and kidneys had already failed. Group A strep pneumonia had started in his right lung, and that side of his chest was filled with fluid. When I examined him he was still awake, although he was unable to speak because of the tube in his airway attaching him to the ventilator. He was so hot with fever that the nurses had laid a cooling blanket over him, a flat plastic device in which cold fluid circulates. The man was a diabetic, and a continuous intravenous infusion of insulin was necessary to control his blood sugar, driven by infection to dangerously high levels. A tube protruded from between his ribs to drain the fluid from his chest cavity. I wrote my observations in his chart: "refractory streptococcal pneumonia, empyema, and sepsis syndrome." He was already on all the right antibiotics; I had nothing further to offer. The trouble wasn't with the treatment; it was with the microbe. Over the next few days his lungs became so leaky that the ventilator machine could no longer supply him with oxygen, and there was little we could do for him.

There's a feeling of helplessness that comes when we can't stop the germ that's tearing its way through a patient. But because I come from a long line of medical workers, my own family stories remind me of how far we've come from the days when strep deaths were the norm.

It was my great-aunt Germaine, a nurse who had worked in hospitals in Belgium and Switzerland, who told me how strep had marked my own family. I visited her when I was twenty-one, listening to her stories in the kitchen of the drafty old house that my great-grandfather had built in the 1880s in the village of Le Sentier, Switzerland, near the French border.

We ate suppers at the little enamel table in Germaine's kitchen, and afterward we would linger, talking. Tante Germaine's gray hair was tied up in a loose bun, and her intelligent blue eyes would get brighter as she got near the climax of the story. Then she would stand up and tell the rest of it from the middle of the kitchen floor, acting out all the parts, but always in her slow, sonorous French, laced with the musical cadences of the Vallée de Joue.

One evening she told me how my great-grandfather, John Golay, brought his new bride, Constance Meylan, to the house on Grand Rue. John Golay, a master watchmaker, was descended from a Huguenot family who had fled across the border into Switzerland. The Meylans were a very old Swiss family, and my grandmother, Lucy, was Constance's first baby.

I can imagine the doctor passing by the long horse trough that used to stand in front of the house and being ushered in through the heavy front door and those thick cement walls that sealed the house in winter but produced a chill all summer long. He climbed the bare stairs to the second floor bedroom where, a few days previously, he had delivered my grandmother.

The doctor would have been unable to recommend treatment for the young woman shivering in the big bed, only confirm the high fever, the dishwater pus draining from the mouth of the tender womb, and the spreading infection engulfing the pelvic organs, accompanied by the intense pain and restless terror of postpartum peritonitis. My great-grandmother had come down with childbed fever, most likely caused by *Streptococcus pyogenes,* the "flesh-eating strep."

Because this infection often spread from the stricken mother to her newborn, the infant Lucy was removed, probably at once, from her father's house and taken down the street to be raised by Constance's maiden sisters, Tante Marie and Tante Berte. Lucy matured into a beautiful but lonely teenager, yearning to live with the brood of half brothers and sisters John Golay had with his second wife. Then group A strep came back into her life a second time, but in a different form. Her illness must have started as an ordinary sore throat, but fever, joint pains, and a rash followed. The illness lengthened from days to weeks and my Swiss aunts called for the doctor. The diagnosis, *le rhumatisme articulaire,* acute rheumatic fever.

Her illness was not related to her mother's childbed fever, which resulted from a direct attack by the streptococcus. Rheumatic fever, which follows streptococcal sore throat, is caused by an indirect attack of group A strep on the human body. In fighting off strep throat, the patient's body manufactures antibodies to the bacteria. Unfortunately, some of these antibodies may also attach to human tissues, triggering a chain reaction in the immune system that causes damage to the host.

Lucy developed the most dreaded complication of rheumatic fever, inflammation of the heart valves. She eventually recovered from the fever and joint pains and returned to school. In 1914 she married and came to the United States, but the slow destruction of her mitral valve, once set in motion, could not be reversed. Her lips were always a little blue, and she couldn't climb the stairs to the second floor of our house in Ohio. The valve in her heart had become tight, the pressure in the lungs had risen behind it, and the oxygen level in her body was chronically low. Lucy was a brave woman and an efficient mother and grandmother. However, she had never known a mother's love, and her inability to express affection saddened my own mother's childhood. All of this was the legacy of two visits by group A strep.

My grandmother's story was a common one, and every time I cleared up a case of group A strep with a simple round of antibiotics, I thought gratefully of how relatively rare such deaths and limited lives had become, at least in the developed world. But there continue to be strep cases that fill me with dread and that mobilize whole teams of doctors, as with Allan Roth, to rescue the patient from an attack by this tiny microbe.

One of my biggest strep battles happened in 1994 when I met Christy Schaffer. She was forty-one and had kidney failure from diabetes. Christy had been successfully treated with a kidney transplant in 1993, and she had been working as a registered nurse at a community hospital in Los Angeles. However, her kidney transplant did not come without a price. Even though a family member had donated Christy's kidney, it was not a perfect match. Christy had to take medication for life to prevent rejection, and these drugs, inevitably, decreased her resistance to infection.

On the evening of February 25, 1994, while at work, she felt feverish and took her temperature; it was 102.9 degrees. The doctor who examined her thought she had the flu. The next day, she continued to have a fever, felt fatigued, and developed pain in her feet. She went to a clinic and was given antibiotic pills to take. Finally, in the early hours of Sunday, February 27, she became severely short of breath. She was taken to a hospital emergency room and then arrived via ambulance to our intensive care unit, accompanied by one of our physicians, Dr. Joseph Kamen.

Dr. Kamen wrote that she was "a large woman who appeared quite ill." The patient was "somnolent" (drowsy) and was breathing almost forty times a minute (the normal rate is less than twenty times a minute). She was in shock, with a blood pressure of 71/45 (normal is 120/80). Her temperature was 101.5. Dr. Kamen heard signs of pneumonia in the right lung and noticed a blister filled with blood on her left index finger. The right foot was slightly swollen and the toes had a purplish color. Compared with the toes on her left foot, those on the right felt abnormally cold.

Christy's chest x-ray confirmed what Dr. Kamen heard with his stethoscope: There was pneumonia of the right lung. Blood tests showed that Christy's transplanted kidney had ceased to function.

He ordered intravenous fluids and dopamine, a medication used to support blood pressure.

Then he paged me to the ICU. "I've got a real sick lady here that I just brought in on a CCT (critical care transport) run," he said over the telephone. "I think she's in septic shock."

Soon I was standing at Christy's bedside with Dr. Kamen. At the academic hospital, where I used to teach, Joe had been one of my best residents. A handsome man in his late thirties with short black hair, a close-cropped beard, and a long straight nose, Joe is married to another physician, and, at that time, his four children were all under the age of five. Resourceful, decisive, and a very good doctor to have around in an emergency, he remembers Christy vividly. "She was the sickest patient I ever transported in an ambulance."

Many microorganisms can cause septic shock in a patient whose immune system is depressed. We discussed the possibilities as I made my examination of Christy. My attention was fixed on the fluid-filled blister on her left index finger. It was about three-quarters of an inch across, extended under the nail, and was filled with maroon fluid. I lifted up Christy's hand and examined the blister more closely. It was deep, but the skin around it appeared normal. This lesion looked like an area of infection that had come out of the blood stream and into the skin.

I figured we'd find our bug there.

I got some Betadine solution to sterilize the skin and a small syringe and a thin needle. Christy was only half-awake by now; it wasn't necessary to give anesthesia. I pushed the needle through the skin covering the blister and drew out some of the fluid. I carefully slipped the plastic cap back on the needle; I didn't want

to jab myself. (It is during recapping that most needle-stick injuries occur.) Then, syringe in hand, I hurried down the back stair-
well to the hospital laboratory.

I bypassed the lab waiting room, which was filled with patients, by entering through a side door leading to the microbiology
area. On my left was a hood with a sliding glass partition that could
be pulled down. A technician was reaching under it and using a
wire loop to inoculate agar plates with specimens of blood, pus,
and urine.

I walked past her to the black slate counter and took a clean
microscope slide out of an open box. I removed the needle from the
syringe and waved my hand over the end to get a whiff of the contents. No particular odor. I squeezed a drop onto the slide. Using a
cotton swab, I smeared the liquid out into a fine film and then tossed
the swab into the red plastic-lined contaminated waste container. I
handed the syringe to the technician with a lab slip asking her to
culture the contents. On the lab counter, a funnel-shaped loop sterilizer glowed orange. I held my slide over the mouth of the sterilizer
until the glass became almost too hot to hold. Now my specimen
was fixed to the glass and wouldn't wash off.

Moving down the counter to the lab sink, I laid the slide on
the staining rack. The metallic sink, once shiny, was purple with
layers of the same crystal violet stain I now poured from a plastic
bottle over the slide. I picked up the slide with a pair of purple-
stained forceps and rinsed it gently with tap water. Next I applied
the orange Gram's iodine and rinsed again. The dried liquid on the
slide was now stained purple. Tilting the slide over the sink, I began
to drip acetone-alcohol on the top edge and watched as the fluid

ran down. When the purple color began to clear, I rinsed the slide under the water, applied a pink counterstain, rinsed again and patted it dry with a paper towel. I now had a Gram's stain smear of the fluid from Christy's skin lesion.

I slipped Christy's slide under the microscope, examined it under low power, and then added a drop of immersion oil to bend and focus the light into the specimen. I flipped the highest power lens into place. Both staphylococci and streptococci, like group A strep, are round bacteria that take up crystal violet on the Gram staining. Under the microscope, there were blue spheres everywhere, in clumps and in chains. I now knew that Christy was in septic shock due to infection with either staph or strep. When microorganisms invade the blood stream, the condition of cardiovascular collapse that often follows is called septic shock. The pumping action of the heart becomes weak, the blood vessels dilate, and the usually brisk blood flow through the organs becomes sluggish. Body tissues do not receive oxygen, and toxic products of metabolism accumulate. I told Joe the news. It was nice to see the look of admiration he gave his old teacher, but it would take more than a quick diagnosis to save Christy.

Christy was now in severe respiratory distress, and she was quickly connected to a ventilator to help her breathe. Her condition had not improved a day later. In my chart note I wrote that she was still in shock despite the infusion of medications to support her blood pressure. Her pulse was rapid, 120 beats per minute. The right foot looked more purple than it had on Sunday. The strep toxins were killing tissues already starved for oxygen, and the abnormal clotting triggered by the superantigen reactions were clogging up the blood supply to Christy's foot, accelerating the process of cell death known as gangrene. In addition, living strep bacteria were still circulating in her blood stream and settling in her skin—there was a new blood-filled blister on her right calf, and another one had formed on the third finger of her left hand.

Christy's husband, James, who'd taken a leave from his job as an electrician to be with her in the hospital, recalled those first terrible days: "The thought of losing her was overwhelming. She's my best friend. I kept asking myself how I was going to raise a five-year-old girl with no mommy. How would I answer her questions if Christy wasn't around?"

For me, Christy was only one of several critically ill patients who had all been admitted to the hospital within a few days of each other. I had a new patient with Valley Fever meningitis, and I was deeply upset about a middle-aged diabetic woman who was becoming rapidly blind from a bacterial infection that had gone from her blood stream into both of her eyes.

I consoled myself as always by spending time with my family whenever I could get away from the hospital. The Monday and Tuesday evening after Christy came to the hospital, Ellen and I planted potato pieces and dried garbanzo beans. As we sat in the garden with the smell of spring all around us, I told Ellen, "These beans are like the ones Jack planted; they look dry and dead, but they are really alive."

By her third day in the hospital, Christy was beginning to improve. She was able to maintain her own blood pressure without dopamine infusions. Her fever was subsiding, but blood tests showed that the septic process was still active.

I finished my morning rounds and returned to my office. For some reason kidney specialists and infectious disease doctors share office space at some of the branch hospitals of our HMO, and my desk was, and is, in the renal clinic. The nephrology nurses all knew Christy, who had spent a great deal of time there both before and after her transplant and was one of their favorite patients. They asked me anxiously about her condition, and I was able to give them a cautiously optimistic report.

When I made rounds in the intensive care unit the next day, I found Christy's husband, James, at her bedside, along with Christy's mother, another constant presence. James had made arrangements for five-year-old Laura to stay with family friends.

Every evening James would join Laura and his friends for dinner. Then he would kiss his daughter goodnight and return to the hospital or home to sleep. One afternoon, about ten days into Christy's illness, James's friends called him at the hospital. "Laura seems upset but she won't talk to us," they told him. When James arrived a short time later, he found Laura curled up in bed crying softly.

"What's wrong, Honey?" Laura did not answer.

"Are you worried about your mommy?" Again she did not answer and continued crying. Finally James asked, "Laura, are you afraid your mommy's going to die?"

"Yes."

"Well, the doctor told me that Mommy's going to be OK."

Laura turned over and looked at her father, "I want to see Mommy."

Christy was still in a coma and was covered with a red, blistering rash. James said, "Your mommy is still sleeping, so you can't see her yet." Satisfied with the information her father had given her, Laura kissed him goodnight and went to sleep.

Group A strep threatens both life and limb: Christy was going to live, but she would lose her right leg. It was turning black as the skin and deeper tissues expired for lack of circulation. On March 2, the vascular surgeon, Dr. Eiji Hashimoto, was called in to consult. Dr. Hashimoto is a calm, middle-aged man of average height, but with large, strong hands. He knows most of the kidney patients well because he is in charge of creating the blood vessel hook-ups used for hemodialysis. A person of few words and no fanfare, he has a dry sense of humor, especially in the operating room. Since dialysis sites are tricky man-made constructions, they can clot up or become infected at unpredictable times, but whatever the hour or day of the week, he comes in and fixes the problem.

Dr. Hashimoto, an excellent general surgeon as well as vascular surgeon, examined Christy's right leg. He noted "non-blanchable dark discoloration" involving the entire foot up to the ankle. There was, however, some blood flow to the outer foot and the fifth toe. It was evident from the straightforward language of his note that Dr. Hashimoto had no hope of saving all of Christy's foot. But perhaps he would be able to do an amputation across the foot, salvaging the heel, so that Christy could walk without a prosthesis.

Two days later I wrote that the patient's pulse was finally under 100, but that her right foot was "cold and blue." For the first time I noted the appearance of a striking scarlet fever rash all over Christy's body. That morning the microbiology laboratory reported that the cultures of skin and sputum were growing group A strep.

Christy's rash was the low point of her illness. In the following days she made a steady, but slow, general recovery. She was able to breathe on her own and was taken off the ventilator. She came out of her coma after two weeks. Like most critically ill patients, Christy had no memory of her first weeks in the hospital. The first thing she can remember saying to James was, "Honey, you need a breath mint!"

"That was on day twenty-two," James says.

Miraculously, Christy's transplanted kidney began to revive. On March 7, I signed off the case, leaving directions to the team to continue antibiotics until surgery was completed on her right foot. On March 12, Dr. Hashimoto ordered applications of Silvadene ointment to the damaged tissue. He wrote that there was "still hope to avoid BKA" (below-the-knee amputation).

On March 16, the nephrologist, Dr. Carlisle, noted that Christy was very depressed. "I knew that my leg was not doing well, but they wouldn't give me a direct answer," she later told me. The physical therapists wanted her to walk on the foot, but she could not. As a registered nurse, Christy recognized at a glance that dry gangrene was affecting her right foot. Dry gangrene is a process of slow death in which an extremity turns hard and black for lack of blood. She kept thinking over and over, "I will never be whole. I can't be a good mother. I won't be able to walk again."

In his March 16 note, Dr. Hashimoto wrote that there was only a small amount of "viable [living] tissue" over the calcaneus [heel] and lateral portion of the foot. It seemed that a below-the-knee amputation was unavoidable. He concluded by saying that he would "start discussion with the patient."

It is never easy to tell someone that they need to have a leg amputated. But with Christy it was different. She was a trained nurse, and she had already decided that her leg was not salvageable. She was ready to be separated from the mortally injured part of herself.

On March 17, Dr. Hashimoto performed a right below-the-knee amputation on Christy under spinal anesthesia. A few days later, Laura visited her mother in the hospital for the first time. James waited until that morning to tell Laura about Christy's leg.

"Laura, your mommy was really sick, and her leg got really sick, so the doctor had to take away her leg."

The five-year-old listened gravely, then asked, "Will they give her a leg to walk with?"

"Yes," said James.

"Then, she'll be all right."

Christy and her five-year-old daughter were reunited after a one-month separation. After a few minutes at Christy's bedside, James asked Laura, "Would you like to go downstairs for a soda?"

"Yes, but I want to see Mommy's leg first."

With some trepidation, James pulled the covers down and showed the little girl the stump. She looked at it with a calm face and then said to her mother, "The doctor will make you a new one and everything will be OK."

By March 21, Dr. Carlisle wrote that Christy was feeling stronger and was able to get into her wheelchair with assistance. She was having pain in her stump and still required hemodialysis, but she was now ready for discharge to a skilled nursing facility for rehabilitation. On March 23, twenty-five days after her admission,

Christy left the hospital. She had a long process of wound healing and training on her new prosthesis ahead of her. At first things seemed to go well, but then Christy's fevers returned. She was worried but initially she couldn't get anyone at the nursing home to take a close look at her. "Finally, I insisted that they send me to the renal clinic."

Dr. Carlisle asked me to come over and examine Christy with him. We found a smoldering infection in her left leg. The skin over the shin was red, firm, and tender. I became convinced that the group A strep infection had returned to her remaining leg, although I could not prove it since her blood cultures remained negative. I was actually angry at this germ that was backing us against a wall. Over the next month, I gave course after course of antibiotics at home, both by vein and by mouth. "I promise I won't let the strep get your other leg," I told Christy.

Little by little the infection cleared. The redness slowly faded, the skin became softer, and the pain resolved. Christy got her prosthesis and was able to walk again.

Since Allan and Christy's illnesses, my colleagues and I have taken care of hundreds of streptococcal infections of the skin and the tissues underneath. The vast majority of patients have gotten better with a course of antibiotics by mouth or by vein. But several times a year a patient will be admitted through the emergency room with a group A strep infection that threatens both life and limb. In many cases, the illness would have been much less severe if the patient had known the warning signs of infection and come to us a day or two earlier. Serious strep infections start out like the flu, with feverishness and body aches. A person may experience a loss of appetite, fatigue, dizziness, and perhaps chills. Simultaneously, or just a few hours later, the individual becomes aware of pain in the skin and adjacent tissue most often in a leg, arm, or the face. Only after the pain is present for several hours does the redness become noticeable. So the tip-offs to a group A strep infection like Allan and Christy's are flu-like symptoms plus pain in the arm, leg, or face, with or without redness of the skin.

Both Allan and Christy have done very well since their life-threatening encounters with the "flesh-eating strep." One morning about two years after her illness, I was passing through our waiting room on the way to my clinic when I saw Christy, who was waiting for an appointment with her nephrologist. Sitting next to her, working on a coloring book, was her daughter, then seven years old. I came over to say "Hello."

"Laura," she said to the little girl, "I want you to meet one of Mommy's doctors. This is Dr. Nagami."

Laura glanced up with a polite smile and a "Hi," and then returned to her coloring. Here was a child sitting next to the most irreplaceable person in her life, her mother. I thought of all the children like my grandma Lucy, left motherless by group A strep. I remembered Lucy's face, sharp and vigilant, and her lonely childhood without a mother. Then it occurred to me that when we saved Christy, we hadn't saved just one life, we had saved two.

a fever from africa

I'm not a traveler. Besides Europe, the most exotic place I ever visited was Marrakech, Morocco. I retain some confused memories of heat, thirst, and Berbers in yellow slippers and white burnooses. I prefer my patients to bring their tropical infections to me. But when I imagine sick people in the Third World countries where my patients travel, I picture them in rural settings, coming to isolated clinics.

Back in 1972, my colleague Claire Panosian, who has always had a special interest in tropical diseases, worked in such a clinic in Limbé, Haiti, one hundred miles from Port-au-Prince but ten hours away by unpaved road. It was a classic Third World mission hospital. Every morning there were one hundred new patients in the concrete-floored waiting room, and every day one or two would die there. The elderly nurses, wise in the ways of triage, always attended first to the babies dehydrated by diarrhea and fevers; then they would assist any adults they could help with the meager resources available.

This type of clinic still exists in poor villages all over the world. The babies with fever and diarrhea are always the same, no matter where the clinic is located. But the diseases of the adults vary. In Brazil, for example, a farmer might seek help for leishmaniasis, a disease transmitted by flies that live in the jungle trees surrounding forest farms. A one-celled protozoan called *Leishmania* is transmitted to humans by the bite of the female sandfly. Special white blood cells, called macrophages, engulf the invaders in the host's skin but are unable to kill them and instead carry the parasites throughout the host's body. In the nose, *Leishmania* causes a disfiguring disease called *espundia* in which the parasite destroys the nasal septum, causing the nose to collapse. In time, the upper lip may become grossly swollen and the palate perforated so the patient can't eat.

In West Africa, adults come to clinics with river blindness or onchocerciasis. The disease is caused by a tiny roundworm and is transmitted by black flies that live along swiftly flowing streams and rivers. The threadlike half-inch long adult females and the smaller males live, often for years, in tangled mating masses in nodules under the skin. The adults do little damage, but the females release two to three hundred tiny baby worms called microfilariae every day. The microfilariae migrate through and under the skin and cause an intense inflammatory reaction that starts as red itchy patches and ends as white leathery skin. If it invades the eye, blindness often results.

In Uganda or Congo, a villager might come into a clinic with a deadly case of Ebola hemorrhagic fever. Ebola is a rare viral infection that appears every few years in remote parts of Africa. Between epidemics the virus probably lives in an animal host, but despite an extensive search its natural host has not been found. The disease was first recognized in 1976, and has caused worldwide alarm because it spreads rapidly from person to person by touch and kills up to 80 percent of its victims. The hallmark of the disease is bleeding, which probably occurs because the virus activates the clotting system and damages tiny blood vessels. Ebola begins with high fever, headache, muscle aches, stomach pain, and diarrhea. Within one week in severe cases, the eyes become red and itchy and the patient vomits blood and has bloody stools. The patient may experience severe pain in the throat and chest, bleeding into the skin, and blinding hemorrhages into the eyes. Finally, the kidneys and liver fail, the blood pressure falls, and the patient dies in shock.

But the traditional village clinic is only a small part of Third World health care now. The process of urbanization is transforming poor countries around the world. In Bangkok, Rio de Janeiro, and Manila, urban sprawl is absorbing millions of the rural poor. Each city has a shanty fringe, sometimes a city in itself. On the outskirts of Manila, thousands of people lived in the world's largest garbage dump, Smoky Mountain. "It was a city tunneled out of garbage," said Dr. Panosian, who visited the site. In this dump, since closed, and in the others that have replaced it, a swelling population of rural refugees and their offspring make a meager living sifting through the garbage for anything salable. They earn just enough to buy a little food from vendors, but not enough to keep chronic malnutrition at bay. Because of this and the lack of sanitation, diarrheal and parasitic infections of all kinds are rampant.

When Americans travel abroad, they worry most about acquiring an infectious disease if they go "into the bush." Tourists want to know what precautions to take on a safari in Kenya, or on a trek to the ruined temples in Cambodia, but they tend to think of hotel accommodations in big cities as refuges from infection. They may not know that Chile's capital, Santiago, is still a good place for a traveler eating a salad to catch typhoid fever. And they forget that in tropical regions, the insects and the serious diseases they transmit don't always respect urban boundaries.

In fact, an increasing number of traditionally rural parasitic diseases are turning up in big cities. Chagas disease, for example, is a protozoan infection that affects the heart and brain and is transmitted by a biting bug called a kissing bug. The bug lives in the cracks and holes in primitive wood, mud, and stone houses in rural areas of Central and South America. Recently, the infection has found its way into big cities all over Latin America, as the kissing bugs have spread to urban housing. Even first class hotels may not provide protection for tourists from insect vectors with wings, as my patient and I were about to find out.

Glenn and I had walked three-quarters of the way up our long block one hot evening in August 1998 when my beeper went off. It was the emergency room. I called back on my cell phone.

The ER doctor said, "I've got a fifty-one-year-old guy here with a high fever, low blood pressure, and a platelet count of fifteen thousand. He's in shock. He's jaundiced and his bilirubin is eleven. He got back from a trip to the Ivory Coast two weeks ago. What do you think is going on?"

"I don't know, but I'm coming in. Would you please ask the hematologist on call to meet me in the ER?" I said.

I walked back to my house as fast as I could, pulled on my work clothes, and jumped into my car. Twenty minutes later I waded through the crowded waiting room and entered the code number to the emergency room. The door swung open and I went in.

It was a typical busy Friday night. In our ER, the fifteen patient rooms surround three counters where the doctors and nurses sit. The usual scene includes paramedics with patients on gurneys, family members leaning over the high counters and talking to doctors, and occasionally police officers filling out reports.

I made my way through all this and plopped down my big infectious diseases book. I had been thinking nonstop about the diagnostic possibilities in this case since I started walking back to my house. The most alarming thing, I thought, was the patient's extremely low platelet count. Only a tenth of the normal number of little clotting elements remained in his blood. Ivory Coast is in equatorial West Africa, and I could think of three viral hemorrhagic (bleeding) fevers that occur there.

The first is dengue hemorrhagic fever, a mosquito-borne disease. My clinical experience with dengue was limited to a pregnant woman who brought it back from a trip home to Thailand. She'd had a low platelet count and a high fever. There's no specific treatment for dengue fever, so we gave her Tylenol and some intravenous fluid in the hospital, and like most patients who receive good hospital care, she recovered. She gave birth to a healthy son about two months later.

The second viral hemorrhagic fever, also transmitted by mosquitoes, is yellow fever. Severely ill patients are jaundiced with yellow eyes and skin because the virus kills liver cells, and bile backs up into the blood stream and skin. As the disease progresses, the damaged blood vessels become leaky and can't contain blood and serum. By then the patient's clotting factors have been consumed, and since the damaged liver cannot manufacture more, bleeding begins. Patients develop red spots of bleeding into the skin and internal organs. They bleed into the stomach and vomit blood. A pregnant woman with the disease would be likely to abort and bleed from the uterus. A hundred years ago they called this disease "yellow jack." Since then we have isolated the causative virus, but there's still no effective treatment. If this patient had yellow fever, he would be my first case.

The third viral hemorrhagic fever I had to consider was Ebola Côte d'Ivoire. In November 1994 a primate researcher working at the Tai National Park in the Ivory Coast came down with Ebola hemorrhagic fever six days after performing an autopsy on a chimpanzee who had died of the disease. The patient was flown home to Switzerland where she recovered. Her virus was discovered to be a new type of Ebola, dubbed Côte d'Ivoire. (It caused such severe illness and high mortality in chimpanzees that they were clearly not the natural hosts.)

All three of these viral hemorrhagic fevers can be transmitted by blood in the hospital. I kept thinking of this man's blood circulating through our big analyzer, wondering how we would decontaminate all those miles of tubing.

I walked over to Dr. Jack Chan to ask how the patient was doing. He was sitting at the counter reserved for the two emergency room doctors. He swiveled around in his chair and gave me the patient's clipboard. Andy Slusar, fifty-one years old, had been brought to the emergency room by his wife at 2:45 that afternoon. His blood pressure had been under 90 (normal is 120), his pulse 140, and he had had a temperature of 101.7 degrees.

"He said it got as high as 104 at home. We ran in a couple liters of saline and his blood pressure came up OK, but with a bilirubin of eleven we think he's hemolyzing."

Bilirubin is a breakdown product of hemoglobin, the oxygen-carrying pigment in red blood cells. When these cells rupture, or hemolyze, the level of bilirubin in the blood rises. (The normal level is 1 mg per deciliter of blood.) Bilirubin also goes up in liver disease—it's the yellow pigment of jaundice. But liver disease didn't seem to be the cause of Andy's high bilirubin, because his other liver tests were only slightly abnormal. So something else was exploding Andy's red blood cells.

The hematology-oncology specialist came in at this point. Dr. Valerie Robson was new to our hospital, and I was meeting her for the first time. She was short and blond, with a cheerful open face and green eyes. She was also about eight months pregnant.

"Listen, Valerie," I said while we were still out of earshot of the patient and his family, "I don't know what this guy has. We're going to put on gowns, masks, and double gloves, but you're just going to watch. Don't touch him. I'm not taking any chances because you're pregnant, OK?"

She nodded in agreement and we stood together outside the patient's room putting on paper gowns, masks covering our noses and mouths, and latex gloves. I slid the glass door open and walked in with Valerie behind me. The patient was lying in bed, his wife in a chair next to him. A male nurse was taking his blood pressure.

They looked up at us, startled by our isolation gear. Andy was a plump, balding man with a weak smile and was as yellow as a yield sign. An infusion of saline dripped in rapidly through an arm IV, and he was receiving oxygen through a pale green plastic tube that ran over his ears and into each nostril.

"Mr. and Mrs. Slusar, I'm Dr. Nagami. I'm a specialist in infectious diseases, and this is Dr. Robson. She's a specialist in blood diseases," I said as we sat down. I had pink progress note sheets on a clipboard with the patient's name and medical record number in the upper right-hand corner. On my consultations, I write down the history of present illness directly as it is narrated. Now, with pen at the ready, I asked Andy to tell me his story.

He spoke very willingly, like a cooperative witness, with a slight Armenian accent. His voice was weak but clear. He'd arrived in the Ivory Coast capital of Abidjan on August 6. He's in the coffee business, and he spent most of his eight days there in a series of meetings. Except for a couple of sightseeing trips by cab, he never left his hotel and had all his meals there.

"Did you get any mosquito bites?" I asked.

"Yes, I think so," he said.

"Did you take any tablets to prevent malaria?"

"No," he answered.

I asked him to tell me about his illness. "It started four days ago, on Monday. I felt a little tired. The next day I went to work, but my whole body hurt and I was still tired. A man who had an appointment with me told me I looked pale. The next day I felt a little better, but my wife took my temperature and it was 100. She told me to stay home from work. Today I felt even worse and my

temperature got up to 104. I had some diarrhea and pains in my abdomen," he continued, pointing to the area below his belly button.

"When I saw he was turning yellow," his wife interrupted, "I
said, 'That's it. You're going to the doctor.' So I brought him in."

I put my clipboard down and stood up to examine the patient, feeling clumsy in my blue paper gown, like a packed lunch.
I couldn't feel much through two layers of gloves, and my glasses
were already steamy over my ill-fitting paper mask. I lowered the
bed rail and looked Andy over for signs of bleeding. I pulled his
lower lids away from his yellow eyes and examined the membranes
for hemorrhage; I looked in his mouth. Then I started going over
his skin. All I found was one little maroon spot of bleeding under
the skin at the tip of one of his toes. Bleeding under the skin causes
these spots called petechiae. In hemorrhagic fevers, like Ebola and
meningococcemia, there will be dozens of them. So, my patient had
a very low platelet count but he was not actively bleeding. Except for
a rapid heart beat and a weak pulse, signs of early shock, the rest of
Andy's examination was normal.

I told Andy and his wife that I was going to examine his
blood under a microscope and that I would come back and discuss
Andy's treatment. Dr. Robson and I left the room and began strip-
ping off our isolation gear. At this point, Andy's nurse came out of
the room, carefully sliding the glass door closed behind him. He
pushed a slip of paper into my hand. It had his name, home telephone number, and employee number written on it.

"Doc, I've been with this patient all afternoon without taking
any special precautions. I need to know what he has. Can you call
me when you know?"

"I'm going down to the lab now and I promise to keep you posted," I answered.

We took the elevator to the basement and entered the clinical laboratory by the side door. The technician had stained thick and thin smears of Andy's blood for malarial parasites, and he now slipped the thin smear under the lens of the two-headed microscope. On the glass slide, a drop of Andy's blood had been spread out with the edge of a second slide into a thin tongue-shaped film and then stained purple. Now, on the stage of the microscope, the lamp shining up from below illuminated a bright violet circle of stained blood. The technician put some immersion oil on the slide to bend the light rays into focus, turned the fine focusing dial, and we stared through the dual binocular eyepieces, which are mounted at right angles to each other.

Andy's red blood cells lay like a field of a thousand flattened jelly donuts. There should have been throngs of blue cell fragments, the platelets, but there were almost none to be seen. At first glance the red cells seemed OK; they were neither abnormally large nor small. And then we saw them: tiny blue rings inside the red cells, each ring set with two red dots. Some of the red cells were parasitized by two of these rings.

I looked up at the technician. "This is falciparum malaria, right?" I estimated that about one red cell in twenty was infected, a rate of 5 percent. In retrospect, I should have done an exact count then and there. I was relieved that my patient didn't have something like Ebola, that I wouldn't have to decontaminate the entire laboratory. I could handle malaria, I thought, even falciparum, the most dangerous type, because I had taken care of patients with it before.

I invited Dr. Robson over to look in the scope, glad to show off my knowledge. In reality, my patient and I were skating on slippery ice, and it was as thin as that blood film, only I didn't realize it yet.

Dr. Robson and I returned to the emergency room. After writing a short consultant's note with guidelines for platelet transfusions, she could go home; her work on this case seemed to be finished. I thanked her for coming in and returned to Andy and his family. To everyone's relief, including the nurse's, I walked into the room this time without isolation gear.

"Andy has malaria and, unless a mosquito flies in here, he's not contagious to anyone," I announced. Then I explained that he had a very serious form of the disease, and that I was going to admit him to the intensive care unit for treatment.

"Do you think that's what Andy's father has, too?" his wife asked me.

"His father?"

"Yes, he went to Africa with Andy, and my mother-in-law took him to the doctor with a fever this evening. She's at the hospital with him now."

I sat down stunned. What would it be like to treat falciparum malaria in an elderly patient? What if there were delays in diagnosis?

"What hospital did she take him to?" I asked.

"St. John's, I think," she answered.

I wrote down Andy's father's name and went to call St. John's ER. "Do you have a Hooshang Slusar in your emergency department?" I asked the clerk who answered the phone. He was there. I identified myself and asked to speak to the doctor taking care of him right away. In a few minutes he came to the phone.

"Are you looking after an elderly man, Hooshang Slusar? I've got his son in our ER. They've both just returned from Africa."

"Really?" the doctor answered, "He didn't tell me that."

"Did he come in with fever?" I asked.

"Yeah, he looks pretty sick," was the reply.

"Well I'll tell you what he has. He's got falciparum malaria. It's all over his son's smear. You need to admit the patient to the intensive care unit and ask for help from one of your ID docs, OK?"

I returned to Andy's room. "It's all taken care of," I said. "I talked to your dad's doctor, Andy. Now I'm going to sit down and write out your orders. We're going to have to give you malaria medicine and check your blood smears to make sure the infection is clearing, so you'll be in the hospital a few days."

He nodded his assent calmly. Both he and his wife seemed reassured and gave me that confident look that is the beginning of the healing process. It's important to instill faith right away, but then you have to earn it.

I sat down at the consultant's counter and opened my textbook to the big chapter on *Plasmodium* species, the cause of the mosquito-borne disease malaria. Until 1999, when West Nile encephalitis killed seven people in New York, Americans thought of mosquitoes as annoying insects that ruin barbecues. But one out of every seventeen people alive today will die of a disease transmitted by the bite of a mosquito. And according to the World Health Organization (WHO), malaria accounts for up to three million of these deaths every year.

The malaria parasite is a single-celled organism, a protozoan. It enters the blood stream through the bite of an infected female

Anopheles mosquito (the males are vegetarians). From the blood stream the immature malaria cells travel to the liver, where they complete their development, then invade the red blood cells. As these parasites complete this part of their life cycle (which lasts from forty-eight to seventy-two hours depending on the species), thousands of red cells explode simultaneously. The body is swamped with the toxic metabolites of the parasites and reacts with high fever, chills, weakness, and shock.

All attempts to eradicate malaria in the Third World have failed. Beginning in 1958 the United States and international agencies began a campaign that promised to eliminate the disease worldwide by 1963. The prevalence of malaria in some areas, such as Sri Lanka, did temporarily decline. Then patients in different parts of the world started coming to clinics with malaria that couldn't be cured with chloroquine, the mainstay of treatment. The malaria protozoan had become resistant to the drug. At the same time, widespread use of DDT in agriculture created races of super-mosquitoes immune to the pesticide.

I would have to base Andy's treatment on where the disease was acquired. In sub-Saharan Africa all falciparum malaria is considered chloroquine-resistant. Sometimes in infectious diseases, however, we can outwit microorganisms by going back to old remedies. So I took out a green order sheet, clicked open my ballpoint, and wrote an order for Jesuit's bark. Not the actual seventeenth-century bark of the Peruvian cinchona tree, but the active ingredient, quinine. My patient would take two quinine tablets every eight hours for seven days. To this ancient remedy I added the old antibiotic tetracycline (doxycycline nowadays), the first dose to be given intravenously and a capsule by mouth twice a day thereafter. In my note I cautioned the admitting family practice residents to be vigilant for two dangerous complications of falciparum malaria: lung edema and cerebral malaria. Then I said good night to Andy and his family and headed home.

The next morning, Saturday, I called the intensive care unit and asked for the nurse taking care of Mr. Slusar. "How's my patient doing?" I asked.

"Really well," she replied. "His fever's down, he ate breakfast, and now he's sitting up watching TV. The residents are planning to transfer him to high acuity."

"Great!" I answered, relieved. "Tell him I'll be in to see him this evening."

I pulled on my jeans and headed over to the Sepulveda Dam Recreation Area near my house. There's a five-mile bike path around it that passes over the Los Angeles River, through a bird sanctuary, and past a golf course. I sat on the open trunk of my old Toyota, put on my helmet, elbow-, wrist-, and kneepads, and set off on my in-line skates to get some exercise.

After lunch Ellen and I went to an upscale department store to spend a birthday gift certificate. She had just turned twelve, and we headed to the makeup counter. I'm a tomboy, but I watched with delight as she shyly asked for advice from the young clerks. As we were walking out to our car, my beeper went off. It was Ted from the laboratory.

"I'm sorry to disturb you, Doctor, but I thought you should know. I'm looking at Mr. Slusar's smear, and 16 percent of his red cells have parasites in them."

"Thanks," I answered, "I'm grateful to you for taking the trouble to call me."

I telephoned the hospital and asked to speak to the medical officer of the day. A few minutes later Thai Nguyen came on the phone. Briefly, I presented Andy's case to him. "I'm working this evening in Urgent Care, and I'll come in early to see Mr. Slusar. In the meantime, could you please run up to the intensive care unit and check on him. Call me back if his condition has changed."

Dr. Nguyen wrote in Andy's chart that he seemed well and had no complaints except for a little trouble looking at bright light. His abdominal pain had resolved, and he had no shortness of breath, although the blood vessels on his latest x-ray were plump with excess fluid. Andy had received a platelet transfusion, but the count had come up only temporarily. Dr. Nguyen decided to give Andy another platelet transfusion and to cancel his transfer out of the ICU.

When I came in at four, Andy looked weak. The nurse said he had barely touched his lunch and his fever had returned; it was almost 103. His heart was racing, but the monitor showed that his systolic blood pressure was a healthy 140. Then, as I sat him up to listen to his lungs, he suddenly collapsed. His pulse became weak, and the monitor showed that his blood pressure had dropped to 90. I laid him down and called his name. He answered me faintly and his speech was slurred. I asked the nurse to give more intravenous fluid and then, shaken, I sat down in front of the computer screen at the counter.

According to Andy's kidney test, the creatinine level had been elevated when he came to the emergency room. I hadn't been too concerned then because he was dehydrated from fever. Now, despite replacement of all the lost fluid, Andy's kidney test was no better.

The British called kidney failure due to malaria "black water fever." Is that what was happening to Andy? I called the lab and asked for the results of his latest smear, which was just being read: 11 percent parasitemia. Maybe my drugs were taking effect, but then why had my patient gone back into shock?

I decided to have a conference with the family. I found ten family members sitting on the circular couch of the ICU waiting room. I sat down and introduced myself. Then I asked how Andy's father was doing at St. John's.

"He's under the care of a young lady infection specialist, like you, a Dr. Joanna Johnson," Andy's wife said. "He looks OK but he is having some trouble with his heart."

I then explained to them how Andy's malaria infection was affecting the various systems of his body. "I think he's going to get a lot sicker before he gets better. He still has a large number of parasites in his blood, and his kidneys are showing signs of strain. I also want you to understand that in the next few days he might need a ventilator to help him breathe."

The family listened attentively. They were as friendly and polite as Andy. Then a diminutive elderly woman began to speak, slowly, and with the same accent as Andy's, but thicker. It was Andy's mother. "Doctor, maybe you should call this young lady who is taking care of my husband."

Plenty of doctors are smarter than I am (my husband, Glenn, comes to mind), but all of my professional life, I've usually known who to listen to and when. This time I listened to Andy's mom. I went back to the ICU and asked the St. John's operator to page Dr. Johnson for me.

She seemed relieved to have someone to talk to. The old man was holding his own. He still had fever, but his parasite count was under 5 percent and stable so far.

"What's going on with his heart?" I asked.

"He's in atrial fibrillation, but I've been able to control his rate."

I told her about Andy and about his high parasite count. Dr. Johnson said, "You know the CDC has a malaria hot line. You should call them right away."

Two minutes later I was ringing the CDC in Atlanta. "This is Dr. Nagami from Los Angeles. I need to speak to the physician on the malaria hot line." The operator rang through to the home of Dr. Holly Williams, who listened to my account of Andy's illness without interrupting.

"Your patient is critically ill," she said. "You've got to begin exchange transfusions right away. If your hospital is not equipped to perform them, you must transfer him tonight to a facility that is. Since he won't be able to take tablets now, you have to convert him to intravenous quinidine." Dr. Williams gave me instructions on how to use the drug, which is toxic to the heart. "I want you to call me anytime, day or night, over the next several days. I'll confer with my colleagues at this end and see if they have anything to add."

I thanked Dr. Williams with a grateful heart, abashed that I had not called her sooner. "There's one more thing, Dr. Nagami. CDC is required by law to conduct an investigation into all deaths due to falciparum malaria that occur in the United States."

I hung up and started thinking madly. Who knows how to do exchange transfusions? They're rarely done nowadays, but I remembered they used to do them on newborn babies with Rh disease.

But how do you drain all the blood out of an adult and replace it with new blood? "Well," I said to myself, "this is a blood problem, so I'm going to call the blood doctor." I paged Dr. Robson.

"Valerie," I said, "have you ever done an exchange transfusion in an adult?"

"Why do you ask?" she said.

"Because my malaria patient is going down the tubes, and the expert from the CDC says I've got to start exchange transfusions right away."

"I'm going to call my chief and find out if there's a machine available we can use. I'll get right back to you."

It was now six o'clock and I was already an hour late for my five-to-nine shift in evening Urgent Care. As I walked down the echoing stairs to the first floor, the horror of the whole situation hit me. "This is an impossible situation," I said to myself. "I have the world's nicest patient with the nicest family. They trusted me and now he's dying of falciparum malaria. I should have called the hot line yesterday. And if I lose him, the CDC is going to investigate, and if that happens, I'm going up to the fifth floor and jumping off."

I walked through the Urgent Care waiting room, apologized to the nurses at the front desk for being late, went to the doctor's room in the back, picked up the next chart in line, and went to see the patient.

At about six-thirty Dr. Robson called me from the ICU. "There's no machine available now for exchange transfusions, so I'm doing the procedure manually."

"Thanks," I said. "I'll alert the blood bank that we're going to need a lot of B-negative blood."

I turned my attention back to the patients in Urgent Care. An hour passed and I decided to go up to the ICU and check on Dr. Robson's progress. Andy was pale, yellow, and almost unresponsive. A unit of plasma was infusing into an arm vein. Dr. Robson was sitting at the bedside surrounded by opened blood donor kits, some with a little blood in the collection bags. She gave me a look of mute appeal.

"How's it going?" I asked.

"I went down to the donor center and got these kits. They had the big needles we needed and the collection bags, but his veins are rupturing and the blood is draining out very slowly."

"It's no wonder, I guess, because he's in shock. I see he's on dopamine now," I said, noting the infusion of the drug we use to support blood pressure. "Let me see what I can do."

I walked out of the patient's room and right into the answer to our problem. It was a tall, husky young doctor I had never seen before. I glanced at his badge: blue university script, bright red border. "Great!" I said to myself. "A UCLA blade."

"Are you on call for surgery?" I asked him. He nodded.

"I've got a little problem I want to discuss with you." I led him to Andy's bedside. "This patient has falciparum malaria and he's not responding to drugs quickly enough. He needs exchange transfusions pronto, and we have to get his blood out fast. Can you put a really big line in a big vein?"

"OK," he said, "but are you sure you want to drain out his blood that fast? He is in shock."

"We'll put red cells and plasma back in as we go, and besides, we have no choice."

A half-hour later, Dr. Robson was sucking Andy's blood out through the biggest surface vein, the femoral, and into an evacuated glass bottle. At the same time, packed red cells and fresh frozen plasma were being squeezed into an arm vein with a blood pump. By eleven o'clock she had removed a quart of blood and replaced it with four units of new red cells. There were big patches of blood on the floor and bright red stains on Andy's sheets. Exhausted from leaning over the patient all those hours, Dr. Robson looked like the spent priestess of some hideous ritual, and Andy looked like a human sacrifice.

The next morning was Sunday. Dr. Robson arrived at the ICU at 7:30. It was shift-change time, when the night nurse sits down at the counter with her replacement and gives a report. Nurses detest being disturbed by doctors at change of shift. Dr. Robson remembered, "I was still new and most of the nurses didn't know me. All of them gave me dirty looks, and when I told them what I needed to do, I got questioning looks, like I was crazy. And I felt crazy, too, draining all this guy's blood out."

By the time I got to work an hour later, Dr. Robson was into her second unit of packed red blood cells, and Andy's blood was draining out steadily from the big catheter in his right groin into a glass vacuum bottle.

"I have to crimp the tube going into the bottle," she explained, "otherwise the blood gets sucked out too fast."

"The percent of red cells parasitized is down to 2 as of 4 A.M.," I said, "so we're heading in the right direction."

"How are you doing, Andy? Are you short of breath?" I asked, as I walked to the other side of the bed and laid a hand on his shoulder. His blood pressure was back in the normal range and he was more alert. But the nurses reported that he had been short of breath all night. Even now, breathing ten liters of oxygen through a facemask, he was panting.

"A little short," he admitted, giving me a weak smile.

Andy's physical examination was deceptively normal. He had no fever, his lungs sounded clear, and his abdomen was soft. But I knew this was the quiet before the storm. Andy had received liters of fluid by vein: saline solutions to support his blood pressure, packed red cells to replace his infected cells, and plasma to replace the plasma we had removed. But his kidneys were failing; his creatinine had climbed to 3.3 and his urine output was not keeping up with what we had to put into him. This is a particularly dangerous situation with falciparum malaria because of the special kind of damage the parasite does.

Of the four species of malaria, only *Plasmodium falciparum* makes the parasitized red blood cells stick to the walls of the host's blood vessels. Normal red blood cells are smooth and flexible enough to squeeze through the tiniest capillaries. But red cells carrying falciparum become sticky and stiff, forming obstructing plugs that starve the tissues for oxygen. The delicate lungs, thus damaged, lose their water seal. The fluid in the blood vessels escapes into the air sacs, especially if there is more of it than the body can eliminate. Andy was now in danger of drowning in the very fluids we had been using to save his life.

It was time to call in more consultants. First I paged the kidney specialist, Dr. John Teague. "I've got a fifty-one-year-old man in the ICU with severe falciparum malaria. He's going into renal failure and fluid overload. Can you give us a hand with management?" I asked.

"Sure, I'll see him," he replied. "Where did he catch malaria?"

"In the Ivory Coast," I said.

Next I was going to need help from cardiology. I wanted them to float a catheter into the right side of Andy's heart so we could measure the fluid pressure in his lungs and his cardiac output. That would take some of the guesswork out of deciding how much or how little fluid to give him. And I wanted advice on managing Andy's quinidine. Too little and his malaria would multiply, too much and his heart could stop beating. The cardiologist agreed to come on board.

Now it was time to check in with Dr. Williams in Atlanta. The results of the 8:30 smear were back. The percent parasitemia was 1.8. Dr. Williams advised us to finish the current round of exchange transfusions and to keep checking Andy's smear every four hours throughout the day. She thought that if the level remained under 5 percent we could stop the exchanges. By eleven, Andy had received four units of cells and had been relieved of another quart of blood. He seemed stable for the moment. I went out to lunch with the family, and then Ellen and I went to the roller rink for a few hours.

As we were on our way home, my beeper went off. It was the hospital, and Dr. Williams was holding on the line.

"Put her through, please," I said.

"Dr. Nagami, I've been conferring with my colleagues at this end. We think you need to resume the exchange transfusions until there are no malarial parasites in your patient's blood smears at all. Otherwise, we think he'll probably relapse."

"OK," I said wearily, wondering how I was going to break the news to Dr. Robson.

"One more thing," Dr. Williams continued. "I leave for Africa tomorrow. You see, there are six of us in the malaria section. Two cover the hot line and the other four are abroad." She gave me the name of the physician who would be taking over for her.

"Thank you for everything you've done to help us," I said, feeling a twinge of separation anxiety.

I paged Dr. Robson with the bad news. She sighed and said, "I'll go right in."

I knew I had to get her some relief or she wasn't going to last long since she was pregnant. By the time I got back to the ICU at 3:40 P.M., Dr. Robson was crouched over Andy again with her tubing and vacuum bottle. I saw a little yellow cable, the Swan-Ganz catheter, sticking into the vein at the crook of his left elbow. The monitor recorded the pressure the catheter was measuring inside Andy's heart. His heart action was strong, but he now required a 100 percent mask with an oxygen-filled reservoir at the bottom, and he was still panting for air.

Despite all of Dr. Robson's efforts, Andy's smear at four o'clock showed no drop in the level of parasites in his blood. It was 2.8 percent. I called Dr. Williams. She told me to check another smear in one hour. At five I went down to the laboratory and peered through the double-headed microscope with the technician. Andy was stuck at 2 percent of red blood cells parasitized with falciparum rings.

Dr. Robson was near the end of her rope. I asked the operator to call the chief of the blood bank at home. He was actually on vacation, but he answered the telephone. I told him my whole sad story.

"I'll come in and see what I can do."

We met in Dr. Burstein's windowless little basement office in the pathology department. He sat down at his desk and pulled out a telephone directory. "There's a private agency that does exchange transfusions using apharesis machines," he said.

"Don't apharesis machines discard the plasma and return the red cells to the patient?" I asked.

"Yeah, but they can jury-rig the tubing, make it run the other way, so that the red cells get dumped and the plasma goes back to the patient."

I waited while Dr. Burstein made some phone calls. It was Sunday evening and people were hard to reach. Finally, he said, "It's all set. They'll come in tonight and do a two-liter exchange. You've got to get a surgeon to put a big plastic catheter into his femoral vein, like for dialysis. Also it's strictly BYOB."

"Say what?"

"Bring your own blood," he answered.

It was about six o'clock when I got back to the ICU. The evening shift of nurses had taken over. Streams of red and white lights from the Ventura Freeway bisected the black rectangle of the window in Andy's room. Dr. Robson had left. Andy was dozing fitfully under a sheet, the oxygen reservoir at the bottom of his mask collapsing and refilling with each breath.

I sat down at the nurse's station and started making phone calls. First to the surgeon to insert a big plastic catheter into Andy's groin. (Not too painful because it could be done through the same hole as the old IV using a guide wire.) Next I called the blood bank and told them they would need to come up with more units of B-negative blood.

"We're almost out down here," the technician said, "but I'll call around the Valley and scrounge some up."

Then I met with Andy's family and told them what we planned to do. Finally I checked Andy's electrocardiogram to make sure the quinidine was not interfering too much with electrical impulses traveling through the heart. Conduction was prolonged, but was still within the tolerable range. I was ready to go home. A little over forty-eight hours earlier, I had never even heard of Andy Slusar. Now I felt as though I had been fighting malaria forever.

By midnight, Andy completed a two-liter exchange on the machine and received another eight units of blood, twenty transfusions since admission. None of the blood in his body was his any more; all of it had once belonged to other people. There were no malarial parasites in Andy's blood smears, not at eight, noon, or ever again. They had been killed by quinidine and doxycycline, and washed away with the blood and plasma of donors. I telephoned the CDC and thanked them. They signed off.

The next day, I was sitting at the nurse's station and writing my morning note, still tired despite a good night's sleep. A family practice resident walked up and leaned over the counter. "I've got a guy who was transferred in last night in a coma with multiple rattlesnake bites on his left arm. The surgeons at the other hospital cut his arm open from shoulder to wrist because of the pressure. What do you think I should do next?" he asked.

I wanted to offer my advice and get involved in the case, but I was so exhausted from my ordeal with Andy that I could only reply, "I think you should call Dr. Sachs. I was on call last week."

We had killed Andy's malarial parasites with drugs and evicted the rest, but the parasites had damaged many of his organs nonetheless. His lungs failed and had to be supported by mechanical ventilation. After a few weeks the ventilator tube inserted through his mouth had to be removed so it wouldn't damage his windpipe, and an opening (a tracheotomy) was made below his voice box to attach him to the machine. Andy's malaria temporarily damaged the hypothalamus, the part of his brain that regulates the salt content of the blood. For several days, his leaky kidneys, unsupported by brain hormones, poured out all the water that his doctors ran in. Lying in a modern ICU, Andy had the serum sodium of a legionnaire crawling across the Sahara desert.

The family practice residents—the pulmonary, renal, and cardiology consultants—took over Andy's care. The ICU nurses came and went, shift after shift, adjusting his intravenous infusions, drawing his blood, and measuring the pressures in his heart. Then one day after more than three weeks in the hospital, Andy's mind cleared. He was breathing on his own by then. He saw his wife and daughter sitting with him. He remembered the doctor had just been telling him, "We're going to exchange your blood."

Then he saw the calendar on the wall opposite his bed. It was turned to September, with a day in the third week circled. "I've lost a month!" he thought. After that Andy made a steady recovery. He began to eat, sit in a chair, and then walk with a cane. On September 25, he was discharged from the hospital and went home. His father had been home from the hospital for over two weeks.

Andy came as close to dying of falciparum malaria as it is possible to do and still survive. Over two thousand years ago the physicians of the Hippocratic School wrote, "Desperate diseases require desperate remedies." Exchanging all the blood of a patient in shock was such a remedy, but it saved Andy's life.

Three weeks after he left the hospital, Andy came to see me in clinic. He said he had a little problem breathing when he exerted himself, but he climbed onto my examination table easily. He was thin, but not gaunt. His blood pressure and pulse were normal, and his tracheotomy wound was almost healed. I gave him a flu shot. He gave me four free passes to Skateland, the perfect gift.

When Andy went to Abidjan he thought he was in a modern city like any other. His taxi took him from the airport to a three-story air-conditioned hotel made of glass and steel. But Andy was in equatorial West Africa.

After a week in the hotel Andy began to feel stifled behind the plate glass. "I wanted some fresh air at night. So the last two nights I slept with the sliding glass door open a few inches. I never saw any mosquitoes in the room, and I didn't even have any itchy bumps," he told me.

"Then how did you know you'd been bitten?" I asked.

"I didn't know for sure, but I thought I had because the last morning after I woke up I looked at the pillowcase; there were five round spots of blood."

manju

The brain is almost two-thirds water by weight and has no moving parts. Its products are intangible: cognition, emotion, and dreams. People didn't always know that consciousness resides in their heads. The ancient Greeks thought that emotions came from the chest. Then in the second century A.D., Galen, a physician and writer, silenced a squealing pig by cutting the nerves to its vocal cords. He followed the nerves back through the skull and discovered that terror comes from the brain.

The brain is so complex that an entire semester was devoted to its study in medical school. The anatomy classes at Yale took place in the old Sterling Hall of Medicine on Cedar Street. We walked upstairs, then around a blue rotunda with gold stars, like a sorcerer's cap, down dark corridors, past old bottles containing two-headed babies and conjoined twins. The smell of formaldehyde grew stronger as we neared the anatomy department.

The gross anatomy lab was a big room with long aluminum tables and deep sinks where body parts, like a detached leg, could be stored upside down. A human being pickled in formaldehyde becomes a dense hulk, the fat under the skin gray grease. Cadavers have a pungent smell, like decaying mothballs that irritate eyes and permeate clothes.

Now, in the second semester of our first year, we had finished gross anatomy forever. The one-legged bodies emptied of organs were lying on their tables under metal covers. We had earned the right to enter the higher realm of neuroanatomy, the study of the human brain.

Fresh brain is softer than a slug; before handling it must be soaked in formaldehyde, becoming a rubbery solid that can be cut into slices to show the gray matter of the nerve cells and the white matter of the nerve tracts. Our professor began by reviewing the structures of the brain using drawings, and then we broke into small groups to compare preserved specimens with the pictures in our textbooks.

On this gloomy winter day in 1973, I picked up an intact human brain, and placing it in the palm of my left hand, I brought it up to my face for a closer look. It was about the size of a cantaloupe. The two halves of the cerebral cortex, the part of the brain that makes us human, were thrown into S-shaped folds separated by deep grooves. As I scanned its surface, turning it this way and that, I was seized by one of the strangest sensations of my life. I realized with a start that I was a brain looking at a brain.

My arms, my legs, my whole body existed only to serve this thing inside my head, which at that moment was directing its left hand to turn the brain so the eye stalks could see it better. My optic nerves were processing the light glistening off the ivory structure. My big brain, life's highest leap, was examining itself at leisure.

That was a medical school moment of detached intellectual delight. But the brain I was holding had once been a real person, with a lifetime of memories. Since then I have had to defend brains under infectious attack, brains inside terrified living patients. Sometimes, as in acute viral encephalitis, the attack is sudden and overwhelming. St. Louis encephalitis virus, like West Nile, is a mosquito-borne infection. It occurs all over the United States in summer months and is especially dangerous in elderly patients. I've seen it destroy the language center of a brain in a few days, leaving the survivor alert but unable to express any of his thoughts with words. I've dealt with parasitic worms whose attack is subtle and insidious. A middle-aged man from Mexico came to the hospital with his first seizure, but his scan showed a brain riddled with grape-sized bladders of the pork tapeworm that had been there for years. Then there's cocci meningitis, an infection that comes on gradually and lasts a lifetime. The things I learned in that neuroanatomy class so long ago allow me to visualize the brain inside the patient's skull, to see in my mind's eye where the fighting is going on and what damage is occurring. But I no longer enjoy the luxury of scientific detachment, because each of these brains has a human face.

One of the most dangerous infectious agents I ever ran into was the smallest, a tiny and imperfect virus. A time bomb set years in the past that was destroying my patient's brain cells while making endless flawed copies of itself. And because adult nerve cells do not divide, once they are destroyed they can never be replaced.

My patient had a rare disease called a slow virus infection of the central nervous system. These patients don't have a "history of

present illness" going back a few days or weeks. Their stories begin
years before we ever meet, as in the case of Manju.

She was small and spindly for eighteen months, and even
though it was December in Chicago, Manju was standing in the
airport terminal in her stockinged feet. She had just come from
India, where baby girl orphans don't always have shoes. Judy, her
adoptive mother, was waiting for her when she arrived from New
Delhi. Her friend Nancy, who worked for Pan Am and could fly for
free, had volunteered to take a week's vacation and bring Judy's new
daughter home.

"I was thirty-one years old when I first thought about adopting a child," Judy told me. "Marriage wasn't happening for me and
time was passing. I couldn't adopt locally. Only severely handi-
capped children were available for single parents. I tried to adopt a
baby through the Vietnam Airlift and from Korea without success.
All my friends told me I was crazy; 'You're single!' they said. I tried
to put the idea out of my mind, but it kept coming back."

Then Judy's friend Diane told her about a friend who was
married to an Indian man. They were unable to have children and
were adopting a baby from the Missionaries of Charity Orphanage
in Calcutta. These people helped Judy contact the orphanage, and
after lengthy negotiations, a baby girl was found for her, three years
into her adoption quest.

I asked Judy whether she had requested a girl. "I wanted to
adopt a girl, yes, but in India, the orphanages are full of girls any-
way. They're the throwaways."

At first Manju was very clingy. She followed Judy's every move
with her large brown eyes and cried if she left her sight. She had

only recently learned to chew, and she was ravenously hungry. In the orphanage all of the children's nutrition had been by bottle. Since her previous medical and immunization histories were unknown, Judy's pediatrician started her shots over from the beginning.

"It was tough at first since most of my friends were single, but I never had second thoughts. Manju was an easy baby."

Judy didn't like the cold weather in Chicago nor did she think it was good for her daughter. One terrible winter weekend the power went out.

"I bundled Manju up so much I can still remember her standing with her arms sticking straight out from her sides. I couldn't get either of my old cars to start at first and I got scared. It was then I decided to move to California."

In August of 1977, when Manju was three years old, she and Judy moved to Playa Del Rey, a suburb south of downtown Los Angeles, and then to an apartment in Mar Vista in West Los Angeles. Judy found a job as a freight forwarder and Manju entered nursery school. Except for one seizure brought on by a fever when she was a baby, Manju was healthy. After the age of six, when she entered the first grade, she was almost never sick and rarely missed a day of school.

When Manju was in the sixth grade, she and her mother moved to Granada Hills in the northern end of the San Fernando Valley. Manju finished her last year of elementary school and then went to the local junior and senior high schools where she was a good student. She planned to work with children as an elementary school teacher.

"By the time she finished her second year of junior college in May of 1995, she had already been working for three years at a local private school," Judy told me. "She was wonderful with children and they adored her. Also, her small size put them at ease." Manju was a little over five feet tall, with short brown hair, a radiant smile that lit up her face, and the same large brown eyes she had had as a baby.

Her illness started gradually. The first symptom happened during finals week that year. She came home after taking her last exam and told Judy that she had had trouble reading the print. "At first I wasn't too worried. School was over for the summer and Manju didn't have much reading to do. I made a mental note to get her eyes checked."

Over the next week, however, Manju had more problems with her vision. It was most prevalent when she tried to read. The lines of print seemed to disappear into holes in her visual fields. Judy became increasingly concerned. On June 6, she took Manju to the Urgent Care Center at our HMO. The nurse on duty checked Manju's vision with the eye chart, and Judy was shocked to learn that her daughter's distance vision was very abnormal: 20/200 in her right eye and 20/100 in her left.

That same day Manju saw an internist and an ophthalmologist. Again she had trouble reading the letters on the eye chart. Her vision was not improved by interposing corrective lenses. In fact, her retinas appeared entirely normal. Could Manju be suffering from an attack of hysteria brought on by the stress of final examinations? Judy didn't think so.

The next day Manju was examined by a neurologist. Neither a panel of blood tests nor an MRI showed anything abnormal. Nor did an electroencephalogram (EEG), which measured the electrical activity of the brain with sensitive electrodes glued to the scalp and brow.

On June 23, Manju's neurologist performed a spinal tap. The count of white blood cells was slightly elevated, as was the protein. These abnormalities were mild, but they were enough to eliminate the possibility of hysteria as the cause of Manju's symptoms. The neurologist thought that Manju might have multiple sclerosis because it often starts with visual problems and it typically attacks young people. He sent a sample of the cerebrospinal fluid for special tests for this disease.

The doctor called Judy and told her that the tests for multiple sclerosis had come back positive. In this degenerative disease of unknown cause, cells within the central nervous system synthesize antibody proteins, called immunoglobulins, at an increased rate. Manju's MS panel had shown "oligoclonal bands" compatible with multiple sclerosis, and her synthesis of the immune globulin called IgG was elevated.

While there is no cure for MS, high doses of cortisone compounds given by vein for a few days can improve specific symptoms, at least temporarily. On June 30, Manju reported to the neurology clinic for the first of three daily infusions of Solumedrol, each to be given over the course of an hour.

"Her vision did seem to improve a little," Judy told me, "but for some reason, I didn't feel satisfied with the diagnosis of multiple sclerosis; call it mother's intuition. I wanted a second opinion from another neurologist in the department."

Manju's appointment with the second neurologist was scheduled for July 27, but by the eighteenth, Judy realized that her daughter's condition was getting worse. She was beginning to have sudden, twitching movements. "She would be taking a drink, for example, and there would be a sudden shake of her hands and she'd spill it."

Judy made a frantic call to neurology. Could Manju come in sooner? The next day, Dr. David Ben-Tzvi, a neurologist in his mid-thirties, saw her in consultation.

Dr. Ben-Tzvi reviewed Manju's symptoms and signs and the results of all the tests that had been done so far. Visual testing with the eye chart in the neurology clinic showed a discouraging 20/200 in each eye. Manju did not have common nearsightedness, in which the shape of the eyeball distorts the focusing power of the lens. Her inability to see was caused by a defect in visual processing in the brain. It could not be corrected with glasses or contact lenses.

Although she did not have any abnormal movements during his examination, Dr. Ben-Tzvi felt that the history was suggestive of muscle spasms called myoclonus, which can be seen in a variety of neurological disorders. Although multiple sclerosis still seemed the most likely diagnosis in a twenty-one-year-old with this kind of sudden visual loss, other diagnoses had to be considered. Could Manju be suffering from a hidden cancer that was producing a toxin or an antibody against the nervous system?

Dr. Ben-Tzvi ordered further blood work and then consulted a colleague by telephone at the Mayo Clinic, who was an expert in paraneoplastic antibody syndromes, as these disorders are called.

"I realized that Dr. Ben-Tzvi still didn't know what was wrong with Manju, but I had confidence in him. He was young and a good listener." In the meantime, Judy had to grapple with her daughter's increasing disabilities. Manju could not leave home and attend Sonoma State University in the fall as she had originally planned. Instead she enrolled in the state university at Northridge, a few miles from their apartment.

"Manju couldn't drive, and she didn't want to take the bus, so she began riding her bike to school. We made arrangements with the disability office at the college for her to have note-takers in her classes. She was only taking two courses, and I went with her the first day to help her find them. It's a big campus."

Then Manju began having trouble finding her way around campus, getting lost from her first to second class. One day she got turned around on her bike and wound up miles from her house. "It was getting really scary," Judy remembers. "My twenty-one-year-old kid couldn't find her way home."

The summer dragged on without a definite diagnosis. Tests for Lyme disease, lupus, and a virus called HTLV-I, a distant cousin of HIV, came back negative. On August 16, Manju went to Dr. Ben-Tzvi's clinic for a follow-up appointment. This time her vision seemed better in her left eye (20/70). Dr. Ben-Tzvi ordered a repeat electroencephalogram to be performed in one month.

On September 20, Manju underwent her second EEG, which was done in a special quiet room in the neurology department. She lay on her back on a comfortable couch while a technician pasted twenty-one gold electrodes in a network of positions over her brain. Recordings were made while she was alert, while her eyes were stimulated by bursts of white light, after she was asked to hyperventilate, and while she slept. The brain waves were recorded on a thick stack of foot-wide graph paper.

As the neurologist examined the tracing he realized with excitement and then chagrin that Manju's EEG now showed an abnormality that pointed to a very rare, very serious disease. Dr. Ben-Tzvi is a quiet man with reddish hair and an athletic build. Like most neurologists, he has a calm and logical demeanor, but I remember the alarm in his voice when he told me about Manju's EEG.

"I'd never seen a case of subacute sclerosing panencephalitis before, but as soon as I saw her tracing, I suspected the diagnosis. In retrospect, the pattern was classic. Every eight to fifteen seconds she had these bursts of electrical activity, each lasting two seconds."

Dr. Ben-Tzvi sent the tracing to our sister facility on Sunset Boulevard for review by a neurologist specializing in the interpretation of EEG tracings. The specialist concurred. If the clinical picture fit, this EEG was highly suggestive of the disease.

Subacute sclerosing panencephalitis, or SSPE, is a slow virus infection of the brain caused by a defective measles virus. Other members of the group include progressive rubella panencephalitis, caused by the German measles virus; kuru, a fatal disease of cannibals in New Guinea; and Creutzfeld-Jakob Disease, a form of the recently recognized "mad cow disease." All of these diseases have two things in common. First, unlike acute encephalitis, West Nile for example, which kills patients in a week or two, these infections usually start years before the first symptoms appear, hence the designation "slow virus infections." Second, the infectious agents causing the illness are defective or unconventional in some way.

SSPE was first described in 1933. The U.S. patients were typically young teenagers living in rural areas, particularly in the southeastern states. Because the disease started with changes in emotion and behavior, the youngsters were thought to be having adolescent adjustment problems. But after several months, trouble with vision, walking, and memory would begin. And within a few years, they slipped into a coma and died. The disease was almost uniformly fatal.

From the beginning, researchers suspected that the illness was some sort of chronic viral infection because microscopic bodies resembling virus particles were visible within the brain cells of the patients at autopsy. However, all attempts to culture a virus from patients with SSPE were unsuccessful until 1969, when three teams of scientists working at different laboratories simultaneously isolated a defective form of the measles virus from the brains of these patients.

SSPE had never been a common complication of measles—it occurred in about one case in a million—but after 1963, with the availability of the measles vaccine, it became extremely rare in the United States. Where it still existed, it was most likely to develop in patients who had had the measles before age four. Manju had never had measles while under Judy's care. If she was suffering from SSPE, then she must have had measles during her first eighteen months of life, while she was still in India. There would have been no specific treatment for this frequently severe illness, but if patients recover there is usually no outward sign that they were infected.

Dr. Ben-Tzvi telephoned Judy. He would need to do a second spinal tap on her daughter. "He told me that he thought she might have a rare disease called SSPE. The EEG was highly suggestive, but he would have to get another sample of spinal fluid to analyze it for antibodies to the measles virus. When I looked up this disease in a medical textbook, my heart sank. The prognosis was absolutely terrible. I decided not to tell Manju anything until the results of the spinal tap came back."

On November 1, Dr. Ben-Tzvi received the results of Manju's measles IgG index test. It showed that the cells in her brain were making antibodies to the measles virus. These results, together with her symptoms and the bizarre patterns on her electroencephalogram, confirmed the diagnosis of SSPE.

"I knew I had to call Manju and Judy and tell them the diagnosis," said Dr. Ben-Tzvi, "but SSPE is such a terrible disease. Most of the patients die within a few years. I wanted to be able to offer them some hope. I knew from my reading that Dr. Michel Philippart, a pediatric neurologist at the University of California Hospital in West Los Angeles, was doing research on SSPE. He was treating patients with interferon alpha, an antiviral agent, so I telephoned him. He concurred with the diagnosis and agreed to see Manju in consultation."

On November 7, 1995, Manju went to the neurology clinic at UCLA. A resident took her history and repeated her neurological examination. Then Dr. Philippart came in with two residents to review the first doctor's findings and to examine Manju himself. Since it is a teaching hospital, Dr. Philippart explained some of the clinical features of SSPE at the bedside. The best hope of influencing the course of the disease, he explained, was to inject the drug interferon alpha directly into the interior of the brain, a procedure that could be safely done using a device called an Ommaya reservoir, the same one used to treat patients with cocci meningitis.

"Dr. Philippart directed his teaching as much to the residents as to us," Judy told me, "and of course, he used a lot of technical terms, so I didn't know at first if Manju was taking it all in. She sat very quietly with a nervous smile on her face. But as we were getting into the car she turned to me and asked, 'Mom, does this mean I'm going to die?'

"I don't remember what I said. It was a terrible moment for us, but Manju didn't cry. Even as a child, she almost never did."

It was about this time that Dr. Ben-Tzvi telephoned me in my office. Would I be willing to do Ommaya injections of interferon twice a week in a patient on an experimental protocol for subacute sclerosing panencephalitis? At first I demurred. "I'm not a pediatrician," I told him.

No, he replied, the patient was very unusual. She was twenty-two years old.

I told Dr. Ben-Tzvi that injecting Manju would be no problem for me. I would just have to arrange the time in my schedule.

I hung up the phone and let out a whoop that could be heard in the next office. "Pam Nagami, former federal employee, rides again!" Here was an opportunity, I thought, to get some breathing time during my hectic clinic days.

"What I'll do," I said to myself, "is demand a full thirty minutes for each injection. Two a week—that's an hour. I can inject an Ommaya in five minutes, no sweat." Even then a little voice in the back of my mind was saying to me, "But this is a tragic case. How long do you figure she'll live? She'll be another one of those dead people in your head you can't get out." I disregarded these thoughts and called up my department administrator.

"It's a very delicate procedure," I said in my most serious voice. "If I rush it, she'll get an infection." The DA (department administrator) agreed to put those wonderful half-hour holes in my schedule as soon as Manju was ready to be injected.

On November 28, Manju was taken to the operating room. The neurosurgeon drilled a hole in her skull, then inserted a small plastic tube through the brain tissue and into the fluid-filled cavity inside. This tube was connected to an inch-long plastic bubble, the Ommaya reservoir, which was then sewn under the skin of the scalp.

On December 4, I met Judy and Manju for the first time. My new patient sat quietly in the big blue chair in my procedure room, listening to her mother tell me the story of her terrible illness and nodding her head in agreement from time to time. Manju answered my questions with short phrases spoken softly through a shy smile. My nurse had recorded her weight on our office scale, ninety-seven pounds. Her skin was dark brown and her eyes large, friendly, and a little sad. Her fine, almost black hair was very shiny and cut in a pageboy. She sat up straight and her neck was delicate, graceful. Manju's quick glances from her mother to me suggested slight nervousness, but otherwise she did not appear afraid. Except for being quiet and stuttering a little over her words, Manju seemed healthy.

Judy was of medium height, chunky, with short gray hair. She spoke calmly, but the intensity of her gaze, and the way she measured each phrase, suggested controlled anguish. Because of my own son's cataracts and his glaucoma, I knew how it felt to sit in a doctor's examination room as a parent. She was a mother to whom the unthinkable was happening. I realized, with a sinking feeling, that I was going to get emotionally involved here, and that what was happening to them was going to happen to me, too.

I stood up to examine Manju's surgical site. The incision was healing nicely. There was still a small bare patch where her hair had been shaved for her operation. I told Manju and Judy that I would keep Manju's hair clipped short over the Ommaya, that it would not be necessary to shave it off again. She could comb the rest of her hair over the spot and the reservoir site would be invisible. There would be no injection today while Manju's incision was still healing.

I walked my new patient and her mother out to the waiting room. Halfway down the hall, Manju suddenly dropped her head and in the blink of an eye recovered with a shudder. It was a my-oclonic jerk, a sudden electrical silence in the brain, interrupting electrical transmission of signals to the body. This was SSPE.

On December 12, Manju came in with Judy for her first injection of interferon alpha. I started with a low dose, 300,000 units, according to Dr. Philippart's protocol. Over two weeks, if Manju tolerated the drug, I was to work up to 500,000 units twice a week. As I injected the cold contents of the syringe through her skin into the little rubber balloon, Manju described the feeling of the liquid entering her brain as a kind of dripping sensation down the outside of her head near the reservoir.

Interferon alpha is a natural antiviral compound harvested from human lymphocytes. Dr. Philippart hoped that it would inhibit the progression of Manju's measles infection by keeping the defective virus from passing from one brain cell to the other. Like many drugs, interferon cannot penetrate into the central nervous system when injected by vein. This is because of the existence of the "blood-brain barrier," a system of tight cell membrane connections that seal off the brain from the blood stream. The only way to be sure that the interferon would reach the site of Manju's slow virus infection was to inject it directly into the cerebrospinal fluid via the Ommaya reservoir.

The evening after the first injection, Manju had a little fever, a frequent side effect of interferon. We found she had less fever if she took Tylenol just before she left the house to come to the hospital. At times during the course of treatment, she experienced nausea, which was of greater concern to her mother and me because Manju had already lost about ten pounds since she had become ill. However, with careful attention paid to her diet and occasional doses of anti-nausea drugs, Manju was able to overcome this side effect as well.

On January 30, 1996, Manju went to the neurology clinic for a follow-up appointment with Dr. Ben-Tzvi. I had been giving her full-dose interferon for over a month. Despite this, Manju was able to name only thirteen animals in one minute. More than twenty-five is normal. She had difficulty doing "serial sevens," in which the patient is asked to subtract seven from one hundred, then seven from that result, and so on. Manju was successful only to ninety-three, after which she made a series of errors. Her vision was 20/50 in each eye. She was unable to accurately copy a drawing of a cube. Dr. Ben-Tzvi wrote, "no improvement on exam, will speak to Dr. Philippart at UCLA."

On February 13, on instructions from UCLA, I increased the dose of interferon from 500,000 to one million units twice a week. That evening my husband and I went to my daughter's elementary school to see her perform in *Peter Pan*. Ellen had been jubilant when she won a part in the chorus. She and I had practiced the tricky songs for weeks, trying to get them right. As I watched her dance in a green leotard, tights, and a tiny skirt of leaves, I could almost believe that she would remain this beautiful fairy forever. But even as I was transported to a magical world of pirates and lost children, I could not wholly forget Judy and her daughter, Manju, who was slipping away to a much more serious never-never land. What would I do if Ellen were to fly away and never come back? I felt a sharp anguish and I said to myself, "You're a fool to play with thoughts like those."

Manju, Judy, and I fell into a twice weekly routine of injections. My nurse would tell me when she had arrived and show her into the procedure room. I would always find Manju sitting primly on the big blue cardiac chair that could be positioned liked a recliner. Her mother sat next to the counter that ran down the right side of the room. In her hand, Judy held the syringe of frozen interferon alpha she had just picked up from the pharmacy. Since it contained only a half-teaspoon of liquid it would be thawed by the time I came in.

While I taped Manju's hair flat, I would ask about her progress. How had she tolerated the last injection? Was there any fever? After feeling for the soft rubber bulb under the skin and clipping the hair over the reservoir with a pair of small scissors (if necessary), I would put on sterile gloves and swab the area with Betadine and alcohol.

After telling Manju I was ready to start, I would pierce the scalp skin and the rubber membrane of the Ommaya reservoir with a very small needle attached to a tiny tube. Judy would unscrew the cap on the syringe and I would take it from her with my right hand. After attaching it to the little tube, I would gently pull back on the syringe to make sure that the end of my needle was in the fluid-filled cavity inside the reservoir. If clear cerebrospinal fluid filled the syringe, I would inject about one-half of the diluted contents. Then I would draw more spinal fluid into the syringe to dilute the interferon further and inject the remainder. After all of the fluid had been injected, I would remove the little needle, dab away any small drops of blood at the puncture site, and remove the paper tape from Manju's hair, which was probably the most painful part of the procedure. Then Manju would stand up and say goodbye, and I would dash off to see my next patient while they took their paperwork to my nurse.

On Friday, April 12, Manju came in for her usual injection but she had a new problem: She was falling periodically. The myoclonic jerking motions, which had started in her head and hands, had moved to her trunk and legs. As she walked, her muscles would contract briefly and then go completely limp, tumbling her down like a bag of bones.

Judy called Dr. Ben-Tzvi, who in turn telephoned Dr. Philippart. The jerking attacks, he explained, were not seizures, though they were caused by a discharge of brain cells that matched the bursts of electrical activity on Manju's electroencephalogram. These bursts interrupt whatever the patient is doing, such as walking or speaking. After a brief contraction of the involved muscles, there is electrical silence. If the patient is speaking, there is a pause. If they are walking, they collapse, sometimes injuring themselves. They remain alert and their thoughts are not interrupted, as they would be in a seizure. On May 14, Dr. Philippart asked me to increase the dose of Manju's interferon to two million units twice a week.

On June 4, Manju had her first two-million unit dose of interferon. Her brain reacted with headache and an alarming fever of

102.6 degrees. Judy called Dr. Ben-Tzvi, and the dose of interferon was decreased to 1.5 million units. On this regimen, Manju had only a low-grade fever after each treatment.

Two weeks later I had a long talk with Judy and Manju about financial matters. Despite interferon treatment, Manju's condition had not improved. She and Judy, who was not working, were living on their savings and on the four hundred dollars Manju received each month in state disability benefits. These short-term benefits would run out after a year. It was a terrible thing, having to discuss long-term disability with a twenty-two-year-old, who just a year ago had been a college student. But I knew from my experience with AIDS patients that applying for long-term Social Security disability benefits was a protracted process, and I didn't want the state benefits to lapse before the federal benefits began. I told Judy that we needed to begin the paperwork.

On Manju's next visit I sent blood and cerebrospinal fluid to a specialty laboratory for a measles immunoglobulin index test, which is a study of how actively the measles virus is reproducing in the brain. The results showed that the virus was not completely suppressed by the treatment, but unfortunately Manju could not tolerate a higher dose of interferon. Rather than becoming accustomed to the 1.5 million units, she was beginning to have temperatures as high as 102 after each of her treatments.

Doctors Ben-Tzvi and Philippart decided to return Manju's dose to one million units twice a week. They also discussed a new medicine called carbamazepine, or Tegretol, with Judy and Manju. Taken orally, it is one of the few drugs that decrease the myoclonic movements of SSPE, but it does have side effects. Because it causes dizziness, the patient has to start on a small amount of the drug and work up to the full dose gradually over a few weeks. In addition, Tegretol can suppress the formation of white blood cells in the bone marrow. Manju would have to have blood drawn regularly while she was on the drug. In early August of 1996, she began taking Tegretol. Fortunately, her myoclonic jerks diminished and with them, her tendency to fall.

During this time, my children finished the fourth and sixth grades and started summer day camp three days a week at a park near my hospital. I dropped them off each morning and picked them up in the evenings after work. On Wednesdays the campers went on outings to local theme parks, and on those days I had constant visions of my kids strapped into a roller coaster hurtling along the tracks at ninety miles an hour.

One afternoon in mid-July I called Manju to give her the results of one of her laboratory tests. She wasn't home. Her answering machine picked up, and I was startled to hear the voice on the other end. She had not always talked in short phrases in a monotone. The Manju I heard on the tape, ebullient and fluent, was a person I had never met.

I left Manju in the hands of her neurosurgeon while I went on a family vacation in August, and when I saw her again late in the month, her condition, while not fundamentally improved, seemed stable. I started talking to her and her mother about the type of volunteer work Manju might be able to do to help with her rehabilitation and to make her life more rewarding. Perhaps she could return to teaching nursery school part time. Judy began making inquiries and a place was found for Manju. It was a happy occasion when I placed a skin test for tuberculosis on Manju's forearm so she could begin working with children. In late September, Judy began to drive Manju to the nursery school on the state university campus a couple of mornings a week. Manju was frail, quiet, and a little unsteady, but the toddlers didn't seem to notice.

On October 8, Manju came to clinic for a routine Ommaya injection with a sore throat. When I looked inside with a light, I could see that her tonsils were enlarged. She didn't have any fever, but I took a throat culture to be on the safe side and gave her a prescription for penicillin. Then I injected the usual dose of interferon.

The following day Judy left me a message. Manju was not feeling well at all. She had vomited once during the night and was unsteady on her feet. I told Judy to bring her into my office right away. When I came into the room, Manju was sitting in the big blue chair. She looked up and gave me a weak smile.

"Do you have a headache?" I asked, concerned that her Ommaya reservoir might have gotten infected.

"No," she answered in a soft voice.

I sent some of the cerebrospinal fluid from the Ommaya for tests to make sure I had not caused an infection during an injection and gave Manju some fluids by vein. I don't think I realized how sick Manju was at this point, even though her speech was a little slurred and she had some trouble understanding what was said to her. I attributed the worsening of her neurological condition to her infection. It never occurred to me that this was the beginning of the end for Manju.

Two days later, Manju began to have really alarming symptoms. She had trouble controlling her swallowing muscles and

choked when she tried to eat or drink. Then she fell and struck her
head on a table and couldn't get up without help. Soon after the
fall, Judy realized that Manju was profoundly weak on the left side
of her body, unable to walk without assistance or even grasp her
mother's hand firmly. Judy telephoned me and I told her to bring
Manju to my clinic to be admitted to the hospital.

Manju was too sick to sit in the blue chair, so the nurses put
her in the gurney bed. My general examination found that her
lungs were clear, her heart rhythm was regular, and, aside from a little soreness from vomiting, her abdominal examination was negative. Manju was alert and could do simple calculations, but her
speech was so slurred and slow that it was difficult to understand. If
she was urged, she was able to lift her left arm off the bed, but she
could not grip me with her hand.

I knew that Manju was being overwhelmed by her SSPE, and
I felt helpless. "Would she have gotten this throat infection if she
had stayed away from the nursery school?" I thought. I pushed
those feelings aside; I needed to know what state of mind Manju
was in.

"Manju," I asked, leaning over the metal side rail of the gurney. "Are you afraid?"

She smiled sadly at me and shook her head no.

Manju was admitted to the high-acuity ward of our hospital.
In my orders, I requested that Judy be allowed to stay with her
daughter day and night if she wished. Dr. Ben-Tzvi examined
Manju, noting severe left-sided weakness. The CT scan of the brain
he ordered to ensure that the tube from her Ommaya reservoir was
in the right place showed no sign that it had moved, and the fluid I

had sent on the previous day showed no sign of bacterial infection. We decided to stop Manju's Ommaya injections in the faint hope that she was having a severe side effect to the medication, but we knew that the most likely explanation for her symptoms was the SSPE itself. The defective measles virus, in its spread from cell to cell, was causing progressive encephalitis, a relentless destruction of the tissue of the brain.

On Sunday, the neurologist found Manju more lethargic still. She did not respond to her name and would move her right arm and leg only in response to a painful stimulus (there was no movement on the left side of her body). Her fever continued.

When I returned to work on Monday, Manju had not improved. Two of Judy's friends from church stayed with Manju while Judy went home to take a shower. I called Dr. Philippart, who explained that, while the interferon alpha treatments had been very effective in a dozen of his SSPE patients, others would enter this sleepy state without warning and not wake up. He told me to resume the injections of interferon, since it was the only therapy we had to offer, and to order an electroencephalogram to help assess the SSPE.

Manju's EEG revealed that she was having powerful electrical discharges every five to ten seconds, the typical bursts of SSPE, but more frequent. The neurologist started the anti-seizure medication Dilantin, hoping that if these excess brain waves could be controlled, Manju might become more alert.

Throughout these first days in the hospital, Judy allowed us to treat her daughter aggressively. We inserted a small plastic tube through one nostril into her stomach to administer her medications, and we gave her nutrition and fluids through her intravenous line.

I was surprised, therefore, when Judy took me aside and told me that she did not have much hope for Manju. After her daughter was diagnosed with SSPE, Judy had talked with several parents of children with the disease. In fact, she knew more about this phase of it than I did. One patient who entered this sleeping state had been maintained for over five years by means of a stomach tube. Judy explained to me quietly that she was not going to let this happen to Manju.

I was taken aback by her clarity and decisiveness. It is usually the doctor who has trouble persuading the family to let go. Judy was several jumps ahead of me, because I had not even brought up the issue of limiting life-support yet. And why not? I asked myself. I had a patient slipping into a coma with a disease all the textbooks said was fatal. Then I realized that I had never expected Manju to die. I had never connected the textbook with the patient. I thought I was going to go on injecting her forever, that she would never stop coming to my clinic; that she was going to get better.

Judy and her daughter, on the other hand, had already discussed what they would do if Manju passed the point of no return with her SSPE. While she was still well, she had made it clear to her mother that she did not want to spend years in a vegetative state. I was stunned by the courage of these two women. Now Judy was determined to be Manju's advocate in the best sense of the word.

By October 16, her sixth day in the hospital, Manju was in a deep coma. Her body was wracked by reflex stretching movements that occurred spontaneously or when she was touched, but she did not respond to her name. The EEG continued to show chaotic unremitting electrical discharges of SSPE. Her short brown hair was matted to her forehead; her wonderful smile had been extinguished.

Her lips protruded or she grimaced, and she clenched her teeth as she writhed. Her unseeing eyes roved under closed or open lids. Inside the dark helmet of her skull, the neural networks of her brain were collapsing as the measles virus continued its destructive spread from one vital nerve center to the next.

Manju never regained consciousness. Her breathing became irregular and she developed pneumonia. At Judy's request we started an infusion of the painkiller morphine. She did not want her daughter to suffer, even in this strange sleep. Each doctor writing in the chart repeated Judy's command: no intubation, no ventilator, and no resuscitation. It is not every day that doctors let a twenty-two-year-old patient expire without putting up a high-technology fight to the finish. Manju passed away peacefully after being in a coma for seven days.

The next day I went into the procedure room and sat in her big blue chair. I looked up through tears into the face of my clinic assistant, who was standing in the doorway crying, too. I stood up and closed the door of the room behind me. I didn't even want to look in there again.

From time to time, Judy visits the clinic. I'm grateful to her for coming in; by doing so, it means she knows I did everything I could to save her daughter. She always sits at the nurse's station in the chair facing the procedure room, and for a long time I wanted to close the door whenever she came so she wouldn't be reminded of all our sessions in there. But finally I realized it was OK to leave it open. Judy and I were ready to remember the year we tried to save Manju, to look into the procedure room and remember her sitting in her big blue chair.

the woman with a worm in her head

Danielle Jordan can talk articulately about her medical adventure now. But on the morning of December 26, 1990, speaking clearly was the one thing she couldn't do.

"I'm not sure what time it started," she says. "It was around ten in the morning, I think, when I first noticed a problem with my speech. It's like I kept losing syllables; they just dropped off the ends of words. When I started losing whole words, I got scared and called up a friend.

"'Jody,' I said, 'would you listen to the way I'm talking?'

"'What about it?' she replied.

"'Just listen. Do you hear anything wrong?'

"I don't remember what I said exactly, but after a while she said, 'You do sound different.'"

Danielle called her husband, Mark. "There's something wrong with my speech. I keep losing words."

He listened to her talk. "I think you had too much sugar yesterday," he said.

"Then around two," she continues, "I drove from our office in Woodland Hills [California] to Simi Valley to talk to a client. I'm in sales and marketing with the phone company—I design ads in the Yellow Pages for businesses. Well, it was about twenty miles on the freeway. I didn't have any trouble at all driving. I could read all the signs, and I found the place OK. It was a florist shop."

"Talking is a big part of my job. I like to ask the clients a lot of questions about their businesses so I can design the right kind of ad for them. We were standing at the counter in the front of the shop. At first everything seemed to be going fine. Then suddenly, I lost my ability to speak. Oh, I knew what I wanted to say, all right. I could even see the words in my head, but I could not make a sound. After a few seconds I heard myself start to talk—baby talk. The client just stared at me.

"The funny thing is, I could still write, though it was sloppy. I frantically scribbled, 'Call my parents,' and their phone number, which I could also remember.

"Just then, the spasm started in my face. It didn't hurt, but it was like a contraction of the muscles on the whole right side below the eyebrow. I was sure I was having a stroke!"

Little by little, Danielle's speech returned. By the time her parents arrived about fifteen minutes later, the spasm was gone and she was speaking slowly but clearly again.

"They decided to take me to the clinic in Simi, and they called my husband; he was there when we arrived."

Danielle told her story to Dr. Diane MacDonald, a family practice physician. She also mentioned to the doctor that her right hand felt cold and her fingers were tingling.

Dr. MacDonald is a large woman in her early forties and an opera fan. When I see her making her rounds at the hospital in her skirts of elegant Italian wool and her sparkling silver jewelry, she looks like a mezzo-soprano on a Manhattan lunch break. Actually, she's a down-to-earth physician with a mind like a steel trap. That day in her clinic she noted that the patient was an "anxious woman, alert and oriented, [who] answers questions appropriately." That is, Danielle knew where she was and was not agitated or psychotic. Danielle's pupils "were equal round reactive to light." So the pathways governing the pupils' light reflex, which travel from the retinas to the brain stem and back, were normal. Dr. MacDonald also noted "extraocular motions intact and fundi benign"—the cranial nerves were moving the eyes normally, and the "fundi" or inside of the eyes, viewed through an oph-thalmoscope, showed no signs of increased pressure inside the brain.

Danielle had a "supple" neck, not the stiff neck of meningitis. The other cranial nerves were intact, and she had normal strength, sensation, gait, and equilibrium.

The only abnormality the doctor noted was that the fingers of Danielle's right hand were slightly colder than the fingers of her left. It was a subtle finding, but it suggested that some recent signal from her brain had altered the circulation of blood to the skin on her right side.

Dr. MacDonald wrote in her assessment that Danielle had been under a great deal of stress recently. She also noted that the patient had a history of migraine headaches, which could be important, since migraine can cause temporary neurological disturbances of all kinds. These symptoms, however, are typically followed by a headache, which Danielle did not have.

Putting everything together, Dr. MacDonald thought that Danielle's history was worrisome, and she wrote, "a left parietal hemispheric lesion must [not] be ruled out." In other words, there might be something wrong with the cerebral cortex on the left side.

Dr. MacDonald had just completed a diagnostic process called neurological localization. She tabulated all of Danielle's symptoms and signs and then deduced the part of the brain from which they came. Each part of the body is controlled by a group of motor nerve cells on the opposite side of the cortex, the outside layers of brain tissue under the skull. The part of Danielle's brain controlling the right side of her face and her right hand were also near the language center of her brain. Based on her examination, Dr. MacDonald knew that if Danielle was suffering from something more than stress, it was going to be a small brain lesion just above and in front of her left ear.

Having gone this far, she telephoned the neurologist on call, Dr. Rasoul Soudmand, and reported her findings to him. He agreed to meet Danielle that evening at the hospital in Woodland Hills, where she went for special x-rays of the brain, called CT scans. Dr. Soudmand put Danielle through his usual meticulous examination. Looking for even the subtlest abnormalities, he saw a slight asymmetry of the right side of the face. It wasn't as severe as a facial droop, but when he asked Danielle to make a forced smile, like a grimace, the muscles on the right side of the face did not contract quite as strongly as the left side. In addition, he noted a mild apraxia of speech. In apraxia the patient forgets how to perform a normally automatic act. From time to time, Danielle seemed to momentarily forget how to speak. She would pause in mid-sentence and search for a word.

Dr. Soudmand ordered a second CT scan of the brain, this time with a special dye that would reveal any abnormalities more clearly. By seven that evening he had the films up on the lighted glass x-ray boxes in the radiology department. The news was very bad, he thought. In Danielle's brain was a "medium size well-defined low density lesion in the left frontal area with [an] enhancing nodule in the center." Dr. Soudmand was fairly sure that this small bright spot on the scan represented a tumor, whose irritating influence was responsible for Danielle's symptoms. In his note he wrote that he could not tell from its appearance whether it was a brain tumor that originated in the brain itself or a metastatic nodule that had migrated there from a cancer hidden somewhere else in Danielle's body, like her breast or intestine.

Dr. Soudmand, himself destined to die of a brain tumor, was then in his forties with thick dark brown hair and a moustache. He spoke with the accent of his native Iran, usually in an earnest, even urgent way. He was not the usual dispassionate neurologist, controlled and detached. His large brown eyes and mobile features showed an almost painful compassion.

On this Wednesday evening, on the most difficult day of Danielle's life, Dr. Soudmand sat down with her and Mark to discuss her scan.

"You have a small lesion in your brain. I don't know exactly what it is yet, but it's on the surface of the left side near the center controlling speech. It's causing little seizures that are making the right side of your face twitch and giving you speech problems."

Dr. Soudmand ordered another scan of the brain, a magnetic resonance imaging study, or MRI, for the following Saturday and gave Danielle prescriptions for two medications—phenobarbital to control her seizures and Decadron to prevent swelling of the brain.

"Most likely," he went on, "you will need surgery to establish an exact diagnosis. I'm arranging an appointment for you with a neurosurgeon." He gave Danielle her prescriptions, shook hands with her and her husband, and said goodbye.

Dr. Soudmand had wisely chosen not to tell Danielle that he thought she had a brain tumor. He left the diagnosis open because he knew that there are limits to what people can process all at once.

Two days later, Danielle was in the office of Dr. Paul Miko, a staff neurosurgeon at our HMO. Dr. Miko was in his late thirties, with short curly black hair, a soft voice, and the sensitive hands of a safecracker. A meticulous person, Dr. Miko takes time to explain things clearly.

He drew Danielle a picture of the pea-sized abnormality in her brain. "It's right near the surface," he said, "and would be very easy to reach surgically. But it's also on top of the speech center, and removing it might damage that area."

Dr. Miko proposed a unique surgical approach. Using local anesthesia, the skull would be opened and the brain exposed. Because the brain itself does not feel pain when it is cut, Danielle would remain awake. Dr. Miko would talk to Danielle as he removed the lesion little by little, checking that her speech remained intact and that the least possible amount of damage would be done.

Dr. Miko then moved to the next step with Danielle; he discussed the diagnostic possibilities. He told her that her lesion could be caused by an infection, like tuberculosis, but that tumor was definitely a concern. He closed the appointment by telling Danielle that he would consult with a neurosurgical colleague at our sister facility on Sunset Boulevard, and he gave her a return appointment on the seventh of January.

Danielle had her MRI the next day. This is a claustrophobic experience, which involves being restrained on a table that slides into the scanner like the drawers in the city morgue. The foot end is left open, but the patient's head is strapped down, and he can't see the open end of the narrow tube. In this particular scanner there was a little glass porthole. Out of the corner of her eye, Danielle could glimpse the technicians in their dimly lit control room.

Danielle's MRI confirmed the findings on her CT scan and showed that the pea-sized lesion was the only abnormality visible in her brain. The neuroradiologist thought that it represented a metastatic tumor from a cancer outside the brain, but he noted that it could also be a glioma, which is a malignant brain tumor.

The following day, Sunday, was Danielle's son's eleventh birthday party, and she was determined to put all talk of illness aside. "It was very important to focus on life and cheer."

In any case, neither Danielle nor her supportive family members make much use of denial. They tend to grapple with problems immediately and try to solve them. So the next day, which was New Year's Eve, Danielle called an oncologist friend and explained her situation to him as fully as she could. He asked for copies of her x-rays so he could show them to a neurosurgical colleague.

That night, the Jordans had a family New Year's Eve party, which Danielle remembers as a happy event. As her parents and friends came to visit, Danielle commanded them sternly "no crying or sad thoughts." She needed to keep her emotions under strict control so she could make the hard decisions that lay ahead.

Danielle's oncologist friend had her x-rays delivered to the neurosurgeon at the university hospital downtown. He, too, felt that Danielle's lesion most likely represented a tumor, although a low-grade infectious process called a granuloma was also possible. He favored taking a tiny biopsy of the lesion under general anesthesia, and if it was a tumor, treating it with radiation. Trying to remove the whole thing, however small, would pose too great a risk to the speech center, he said.

Danielle's oncologist friend thought that further neurosurgical opinions were needed, as this seemed to be an area of therapeutic controversy. He sent the x-rays to a neurosurgeon in Toronto, Canada, who specialized in cortical mapping surgery in patients while awake, like the surgery Dr. Miko had proposed. The surgeon made a little conference of Danielle's case by showing her films to three of his colleagues. On January 10, the Canadian neurosurgeon called with his assessment of Danielle's situation. This was most likely a primary brain tumor called a glioma. He agreed with the university surgeon: Biopsy the lesion and treat with radiation depending on the final pathology.

Four days later, Danielle had a consultation with a surgeon at a hospital in Los Angeles who was also a well-known authority on cortical mapping neurosurgery. Danielle felt that his manner was both blunt and devastating. "He told me I had a very bad brain tumor and that I had only a 50 percent chance of being alive in three years."

Danielle's husband and parents were present, and her mother felt faint. When Danielle returned home from the appointment, her two sons saw her crying, and, for the first time, they thought their mother might die.

Danielle was now at the psychological low point of her ordeal, but her luck was about to change. One of Danielle's friends got in touch with the wife of a neurosurgeon at the University of California in Irvine, Dr. Leslie Cahan. Dr. Cahan invited Danielle to bring her x-rays to his house after he returned home from his long workday. At ten o'clock that evening, Danielle and her family met with Dr. Cahan around his dining room table. Dr. Cahan lifted the films up to the light and exclaimed, "I don't see a tumor. I see cysticercosis, a kind of worm."

Dr. Cahan's wife screamed happily and hugged Danielle. "My husband is brilliant. He'd never say it if he weren't sure."

What Danielle Jordan had just been told was that she was the host of the pork tapeworm. Dr. Cahan thought the pea-shaped abnormality in her brain was a larval worm.

Where did it come from? Since Danielle was an observant Jewish woman, it was unlikely that she'd gotten it by eating undercooked infected (measly) pork. Since antiquity, people have seen the pea-sized cysts, called bladders, in pig muscles. (Aristotle thought they made the meat tender.) These bladders, or cysticerci, are the encysted larvae of the pork tapeworm, *Taenia solium*. If you make a meal of such pork, and the larvae haven't been killed by thorough cooking, they're released from the meat during digestion and attach to the wall of the small bowel by little hooks. The tapeworm may eventually grow to be over three yards long, but because it is very thin and flat, it usually doesn't cause any symptoms.

The worm settles in for what may be a ten-year lifespan, and over that time it tries to reproduce by fertilizing its own eggs (it's a hermaphrodite), which are neatly packaged in segments that fall off the end of the worm and are passed in the stool. Twenty to thirty thousand eggs go into the stool every day, and those tiny eggs become the source of more infections.

They may, in the Third World, infect a pig that's foraging near a leaking privy or in a field where human waste is used as fertilizer. Or they may infect humans who eat raw food, such as salads or fruit that has come in contact with soil contaminated by sewage. It's also possible for a human carrier of an adult tapeworm to contaminate food while preparing it. The worm's minute eggs pass from the intestines to toilet paper, to unwashed hands, to the surface of food, and into the body of a new host.

If a person eats a tapeworm egg, the shell around the egg is digested in the stomach and a living embryo, called an oncosphere, is released. Oncospheres are able to penetrate the wall of the intestine and are carried by the blood stream all over the body of the intermediate host. They can settle anywhere, but are most often found in the muscles, the brain, and the eye. In these locations, the oncospheres grow, and after sixty to seventy days, they are mature bladder worms (like the cysts in measly pork) called cysticerci. Each cysticercus larva has eight little hooks and four suckers at the head end. If Dr. Cahan's hypothesis was correct, Danielle Jordan had somehow eaten the egg or eggs of a pork tapeworm, which then found a home in her brain and developed into a tiny larval worm.

Cysticercosis is not rare. In fact, it's the most common parasitic infection of the brain, and, based on the total number of patients affected, it is the most frequent cause of seizures worldwide. Why hadn't the other doctors considered this diagnosis?

"I was the victim of my own last name," Danielle says. "If I'd had a Hispanic name, someone would have thought of cysticercosis, I think. In fact, when Dr. Cahan showed my films to several of his colleagues at Irvine, without telling them my history, most of them thought that I had cysticercosis, too." But outside of Southern California and other areas with large populations of Hispanic immigrants, doctors don't expect to see cysticercosis.

In neurocysticercosis, it is not uncommon for a patient's brain to be riddled with a dozen quarter-inch holes, each the home of a dormant worm. But if Danielle had the disease, her prognosis should be excellent because her scans showed only one lesion. So Danielle had reason for hope, but she still did not have a definite diagnosis. Of course, her neurosurgeon, Dr. Miko, could perform a biopsy, but whether it was a tumor or a worm, Danielle's lesion was still sitting directly on top of her speech center. Any surgical procedure could result in permanent damage to that area.

On January 17, Dr. Miko performed a spinal tap on Danielle. He sent samples of her cerebrospinal fluid and blood to a laboratory to be analyzed for antibodies to *Taenia solium*, the pork tapeworm. The next day, Danielle came to my office for an infectious disease consultation. She told me her whole history, from the time she fell out of a window at the age of three, suffering a concussion, through her recent nerve-wracking series of neurosurgical consultations.

Danielle had been born and raised in New York and had moved to California at age six. Three years previously, she and her husband had purchased a time-share condominium in Cancún, but they had been regular travelers to Mexico, a high-risk area for cysticercosis, for many years before that.

"Danielle," I said, "I think you probably have cysticercosis, but you must understand that the tests are not 100 percent exact. You may not be sure of what you have for months. Even if I give you medicine to kill the worm, your scan may not change. Dr. Miko can operate right away and put an end to this uncertainty, but you already know the risks of surgery."

I looked at the intelligent face of the woman sitting across from me. She was slim, in her early forties, stylishly put together—clothes, hair, nails—the successful salesperson. But when her speech had failed that morning without warning, and when her scans had shown that lesion, I knew she had had to face her own mortality. Now she had the steady look of a soldier hunkered down in a foxhole, and I remember thinking she was someone who knows that fear alone can't kill you. So I wasn't surprised when she decided to go with medical therapy, even if it meant living for months without knowing whether she had a tumor in her brain or a worm.

"If this is cysticercosis, Doctor, how long do you think I've had it?" Danielle asked.

"The chances are that you've been harboring this worm for at least six years. First of all, it takes time for it to get this big" (and to grow those suckers and hooks, I thought to myself). "The amazing thing about this parasite is that as long as it's healthy the immune system doesn't seem to know it's there. The larval worm secretes something that puts the inflammatory reaction to sleep like a drugged watchdog. It also controls the amount of fluid passing across the cyst membranes from the brain.

"Then, anywhere from six to ten years or more after you're infected, the little worm gets tired of waiting for a predator to eat you and it dies. That's when the trouble starts. The immune cells wake up and try to devour the parasite with enzymes. The dying wall around the worm stops regulating how much fluid gets in and the cyst starts to swell. The brain becomes irritated and you have seizures. Living worms can take up space and cause problems, don't get me wrong, but in the form of the disease I think you have, it's the dying worm that's making you sick."

"If the worm's already dying, why do I need medicine to kill it?" Danielle asked.

"You may have other cysticerci in your body that are still alive. It's unusual to ingest only one egg. Also, some authorities think that the worm dies gradually and that medicine speeds up the process and leads to a better outcome."

I made Danielle an appointment to see me on January 22, and I said goodbye with an upbeat smile and a confident handshake. I remember thinking to myself after she left, "What if that blood test comes back negative, then what?" I like to believe that I heal patients by taking control and projecting competence. But I had biased Danielle in the direction of a curable infectious disease. What if I was wrong, carried away by my tendency to see the whole world as infected with something or other?

It was ironic that Danielle, who was forbidden by her religion to eat pork, should find herself host to a pork tapeworm larva, but it wasn't too surprising that she'd picked up some sort of parasite. We all have them. The pneumocystis organisms that cause pneumonia in patients with AIDS, for example, live quietly in everyone's lung as a commensal species that "eats at our table" (as the name means) without harming us. But when the immune system fails, they start to multiply and become harmful parasites. In the natural world, parasitic species outnumber free-living ones two to one—parasitism is universal. And in parts of the world where human waste cycles through the environment, everyone is host to several species of worms.

Danielle's appointment was in the morning. According to my diary, by the time I got home that Friday night, I was preoccupied not with parasites, but with the burden of work in my office. Besides my infectious disease consultations, I'm the personal physician to my patients at the HMO, twenty of whom might call me on an average day with problems ranging from a runny nose to chest pain. Each cholesterol test I order and every Pap smear I do has to be followed up. Fridays can be very discouraging, because after working hard all week, the pile of lab tests, x-ray reports, and messages on my desk seems higher than ever. That particular week I'd been a real hamster on a wheel.

On Saturday morning, I got up, still tired, and went to the hospital to make rounds. An hour or so later, while I was seeing patients, my beeper went off. It was my husband, Glenn.

"Ellen has an earache," he said.

I saw another patient, then went down to the Urgent Care Center to meet my family, who had driven the seven miles from our house to the hospital. Ellen was sitting quietly on Glenn's lap, her brown hair obscuring her father's face. I made sure they were checked in OK; then I went back upstairs to finish my rounds. I was working in the intensive care unit when the nurse ran out of one of the rooms and called a code blue. A three-year-old girl with leukemia had gone into cardiac arrest. Moments later, a pediatrician sprinted in from Urgent Care on his way to the code.

"Your daughter has otitis in both ears, right worse than the left," he shouted at me as he ran by and into room three.

"Damn!" I said, mortified with myself. Ellen had had a cold and an earache since Thursday, and I should've brought her in sooner.

Through the open door of room three, I could see the pediatrician frantically trying to resuscitate the little girl. I looked away. I didn't like to think about anyone's kid being that sick.

I awoke in the small hours of Sunday morning from a nightmare that I don't remember. A few hours later, I was back in intensive care making Sunday morning rounds. Someone else was in the room where the little girl had been.

When I got home around lunchtime Ellen looked like her old self. In the afternoon the kids and I made three bowls of "soup" using leaves and flowers we found outside for seasoning. I hugged both children and I took their pictures.

January 22 came, and to my infinite relief, Danielle's serum cysticercosis test was positive. As it turned out, the neurosurgeon at our own sister facility at Sunset Boulevard, after independently reviewing Danielle's films, was also considering the diagnosis of neurocysticercosis, so it's unlikely that she would have been subjected to unnecessary surgery, even if she had not sought outside opinions. But what Danielle had done was sound. She'd sensed that her condition was complex and controversial, and she didn't hesitate to pool the knowledge of several physicians.

Now it was time to discuss treatment. An ophthalmologist would check for larval worms in her eyes, because killing them suddenly could cause enough inflammation to produce permanent damage to her vision. Then she'd spend a few days in the hospital while receiving the first round of anti-worm drugs, in case the dying parasite in her brain caused an increase in her seizures. And finally, she'd be taking Decadron, a corticosteroid medication, to minimize the amount of brain swelling the parasite would cause. This last decision was the most controversial, because Decadron would also decrease the concentration of the worm medicine in her brain, and could lead to treatment failure. It was worth the risk, though—we didn't want to allow undue inflammation in her speech center when the worm finally died.

Everything went smoothly. The ophthalmologist examined her eye from lens to retina and found no worms, so on February 4, Danielle was admitted to the hospital. An intravenous line was inserted in case of seizures, and she received her first Decadron pill along with the worm-killer, praziquantel. I had x-rays taken of her thighs, looking for round calcium deposits that might be left by old worm larvae—there were none—and sent a sample of her blood to the state laboratory for confirmatory tests for cysticercosis.

One day into her treatment, Danielle began to have a mild headache and the next day she had a low-grade fever. It looked like I was getting a reaction from Danielle's worm, a sign that my treatment was working.

The following day Danielle felt better, and the day after that she went home. She would need to take praziquantel tablets three times a day for a total of fifteen days. On February 13 she came to my clinic for an appointment. She was seven days into her treatment and she felt fine.

Danielle finished her praziquantel on February 22. For two days near the end, she again had a slight headache and then felt well. About two weeks later she had another magnetic resonance scan of her brain; the swelling had resolved completely. The only evidence of her "tumor" was "a very small focus of enhancement in the convexity of the left posterior frontal lobe." It was the dying worm flickering out like a candle.

In early April, I received a letter from the Reference Immuno-diagnostic Laboratory, Parasitic Diseases Branch of the Centers for Disease Control. Danielle's blood had made it from the state lab all the way to Atlanta, Georgia. Her immunoblot assay was positive for cysticercosis. Would I please return the enclosed case report form? After they received my report, I remember discussing the case with the doctors there by telephone. They were delighted that their new test had registered a positive in a patient with just one worm. I'm always happy to talk to the people at CDC, the mecca of infection.

Shortly thereafter, the Los Angeles County Health Department called. They had learned about Danielle's case, probably through the state lab. Would I please obtain stool specimens for ova and parasites from Danielle's two sons and her husband and send the results? (Danielle's had already been submitted and was negative.) These samples were also negative.

Danielle was able to return to work in early May 1991, although she still had bouts of mild right facial twitching from time to time through that spring. A final brain MRI done in April 1994 showed only a tiny, two-millimeter abnormality, Danielle's souvenir of her encounter with a little worm.

Danielle had parenchymal neurocysticercosis. A tapeworm egg that got into her blood stream lodged in the parenchyma or substance of her brain. In patients with severe cases of this form of neurocysticercosis, the brain can look exactly like a piece of Swiss cheese. I trace my earliest interest in science to two ghastly pictures in my mother's college textbook, *Animals Without Backbones* by Ralph Buchsbaum. The first photograph showed the formalin-fixed brain of a patient who had died of neurocysticercosis. It was sliced in half and had so many grape-sized bladders in it that it was a wonder that the patient had lived long enough for all of them to grow to that size. (The other picture was the grotesquely swollen right leg of a patient with elephantiasis from a tropical worm.)

Except in extreme cases, like the one in my mother's textbook, the prognosis of parenchymal neurocysticercosis is relatively favorable. In the mid-1990s, albendazole became available in the United States and is now the drug of choice for the disease. Like praziquantel, it can be given by mouth, but it has two advantages over the older drug: It is more reliably concentrated in the brain and is better at killing the parasitic worm.

In the years since Danielle came to me with her cysticercosis, other parasites have crossed my path: malaria, bladder flukes, and roundworms eight inches long. But no one since Danielle, who thought she had a brain tumor, has ever been so happy to have a worm.

I still give my kids extra hugs when bad things happen at work, even though my son is now taller than I am. The pages of my diary are my video camera. I ask my children, "Do you remember the time we made soup from leaves and flowers?"

"Soup? No, Mom," they answer.

"Ellen, do you remember when Daddy brought you in with an ear infection and I met you in Urgent Care?"

"I had lots of ear infections," she replies.

Memory is a funny thing. Danielle Jordan says that it wasn't until I took her history that she remembered how and when she probably caught her cysticercosis.

"I'd forgotten all about that lunch in Puerta Vallarta, until you started asking me questions. It was in December, six or seven years before I got sick. We went with another family to a famous restaurant where all the movie stars go. You can't drive to it; you have to walk. I'd been traveling in Mexico for years and I should have known better, but that day I did something I would never have done ordinarily."

"What was that?" I asked.

"I ordered salad."

chapter 9

septic shock

Most people think of life-threatening infections as rare catastrophes that happen to someone else. We're not likely to sample raw snake, and HIV is something we hope to avoid. But there is one syndrome, septic shock, that can happen to anyone. Septic shock is the roller-coaster drop in blood pressure that follows blood stream invasion by germs. Frequently, the lungs, kidneys, and other organs also fail. Although viruses and fungi can cause the syndrome, the most common cause is bacteria. In the United States, between fifteen and twenty thousand people die of the syndrome every year.

Whether the source of the infection is obvious, or hidden, as in the following story, the process moves with lightning speed.

I was sitting in the basement of the hospital listening to a lecture and eating a cookie one Tuesday afternoon when my beeper went off.

"We have a patient of yours in the emergency room, Doris Silver. Do you remember her?" asked the doctor over the telephone.

"Yes," I answered. Doris was a grandmotherly woman in her sixties who recently had part of her colon removed for cancer. She was still receiving chemotherapy, and I had been assigned to be her primary care physician.

Doris, the ER doc told me, was in shock. She'd been sick for four days, and now her blood pressure was low and dropping. "It started with weakness," the doctor said, "then on Sunday she came to the ER a little confused. The lab tests and brain CT were normal so they sent her out on oral antibiotics. But today her family says she's been delirious and falling down. I think she's septic. I'm trying to get her blood pressure up with dopamine now, and we're admitting her to the ICU."

"I'll be right there," I said, and hung up the phone.

Septic shock is the ultimate infectious disease emergency. Although I've been dealing with it all of my professional life, it's never routine. Each patient with the syndrome presents a unique set of life-threatening symptoms and signs and gets added to my mental file of patients. One patient was brought in with high fever and low blood pressure after collapsing in a hotel bathroom. She'd had her spleen removed after a car accident ten years before and, robbed of this first line of defense against blood stream invasion, she died in less than twelve hours from pneumococcus, a kind of strep. Then there was the patient with cirrhosis of the liver who had arrived at the walk-in clinic feeling sick after swimming in the ocean. I remembered him crashing in the ICU with a strange salt-water bacterium called a Vibrio that raised big welts on his legs. It was just starting to show up in his blood cultures when he died three days later. And I'll never forget the young woman who had gas gangrene on her left leg. By the time we got her to the operating room, she had all the signs of septic shock: low blood pressure, delirium, and no clotting factors. When the surgeon cut her leg open her muscles looked like meat reduced for a quick sale. I can still hear the cellophane wrap crinkle of gas bubbles under her skin and smell the sickly sweet pus that oozed out of her wound.

Septic shock is a bolt out of the blue that can strike anyone, but elderly patients, like Doris, are the most frequent victims. People are living longer with a variety of chronic conditions that make them susceptible to serious infections. Diabetics go septic when their kidneys or feet get infected. Patients with heart and lung disease get into trouble with pneumonia. And people go into shock following surgical procedures on germ-filled intestines. Some of the most dangerous blood infections follow chemotherapy because it leaves the patients' immune systems vulnerable to bacterial invasion. That's what I figured was happening with Doris. Her septic shock was somehow related to her chemotherapy for colon cancer.

Cases like Doris's were one of the reasons my first year at the HMO had been so difficult for me. At the VA, where I worked for seven years between my last fellowship and my job at the HMO, the residents I supervised always stood between the patient and me. They were the ones who did the night calls. They performed the invasive procedures like putting tubes down patients' airways and hooking them up to ventilators. I was the armchair quarterback who critiqued their work.

But at the HMO I had to face the patient directly, make on-the-spot decisions and then stand behind them. I worried that my knowledge was rusty or out-of-date. I wasn't as confident as I would have liked to have been about the little details of care, like exactly how much insulin a diabetic should get or how to adjust a ventilator. I was always afraid someone might question my orders.

In the evenings Glenn and I would sit at our kitchen table, drinking decaf, and I would tell him about all the trouble I was having at my new job.

"They're going to find out I'm a fraud!" I said after one really bad day.

My husband likes to make a game of misunderstanding me. He says I have a Great Lakes accent.

"Why will they find out you're a frog?" he asks.

"Fraud, Glenn, that I don't know anything," I said. But fraud, frog—I felt like both.

Now, in my first year on the job, one of the things that kept me going was the oasis in my schedule on Tuesday afternoons. There would be a special lunch, and in the afternoon, instead of seeing patients, the internists and family medicine doctors had lectures and refreshments. We all lived for these breaks, but they were often punctuated by the sound of a beeper followed by chairs scraping and whispered apologies as one of the doctors made a hasty exit. It was during one of these lectures that I got the call about Doris.

When I got there, Doris's nurse was getting ready to move her to the ICU on the second floor. She disconnected her facemask tubing from the wall oxygen and connected it to a portable tank. She transferred the heart leads from the wall monitor to a small unit on Doris's gurney. An infusion pump mounted on a rolling pole regulated the flow of saline solution and the blood pressure supporter, dopamine.

Doris's forty-one-year-old son, Jonathan, was at her bedside. His younger sister, Sharon, arrived just after I did. She was thin, with alert brown eyes that took in everything. While her brother was quiet and reserved, Sharon was lively and full of questions.

"I'm so glad to see you!" she said, rushing up to me. "My mother told me how you took care of her when she was in the hospital and she has so much faith in you."

I managed a wan smile. My patient was only semiconscious and she was breathing fast. "Your mom's pretty sick now. Can you tell me what happened today?"

"She went to temple for services with a couple of her friends," Sharon said.

I remembered then that it was Yom Kippur, the Day of Atonement. In my ultra-reformed Jewish childhood, we practiced Yom Kippur-lite—we stayed home from school.

"Did she fast?" I asked.

"No, she didn't because of her chemotherapy, but they had been there since this morning and I don't think they had lunch. Her friends said she seemed groggy and unsteady on her feet, so they took her to my brother's house. A little while later Jonathan's wife found her on the bathroom floor and she called 911."

The ER nurse signaled me that she was ready to move the patient. I took up my position at the foot end of the gurney.

When we arrived in the ICU we were motioned to a single room and the receiving nurse and the ER nurse deftly moved Doris onto the waiting bed by picking up the ends of the sheet she was lying on. The ICU nurse, a tall thin man in blue scrubs, leaned over Doris to plug her oxygen line into the wall. Then he turned on the lights of her monitor and transferred the leads from the portable unit. I introduced myself and he gave me a quick but friendly smile and told me his name was Alex. He had a very slight stutter that made him seem shy, but his hands moved with a competence I envied.

Alex wrapped a blood pressure cuff around Doris's upper arm and pumped it up. "What's her BP?" I asked.

"Eighty-six over fifty," he said. Then he gave me a full report on her pulse, temperature, respiration, oxygen flow, and IVs.

Although Doris did not have much fever, her blood count was alarming. Sixty-four percent of her white blood cells were band forms. These are the immature white cells that get pushed out of the bone marrow before their time during really serious infections. Ten percent bands is a lot; sixty percent suggests an overwhelming invasion of the blood stream. People are familiar with the term *antiseptic*. But the positive term, sepsis, is what the antiseptics are trying to protect us from. And Doris had all the signs of sepsis. Besides her low blood pressure and high white count, she had an ominously low platelet count of only seventy thousand, which was about half of normal. Platelets are the cell fragments that help the blood to clot. But bacterial toxins in the blood stream activate platelets as well and cause them to be uselessly consumed.

All of these abnormalities of the blood tend to be more severe in septic cancer chemotherapy patients because the bone marrow factory that produces the blood elements as they are consumed is impaired by chemotherapy. Chemotherapy agents target the rapidly dividing cancer cells, but the blood-making cells in the bone marrow are also rapidly dividing, which is why they come in for so much damage.

I remember one infected patient with lymphoma whose platelet count dropped so low that he started bleeding into his lungs. Blood welled up into his ventilator tubing and threatened to drown him. Another terrible complication of a low platelet count is bleeding into the brain, which can happen without warning. Within the tight confines of the skull, there's nowhere for this blood to go. It can crush brain tissue and kill the patient in a few hours.

So I had to get Doris's infection under control and stop the destructive process in the blood stream before it got any worse. I ordered blood cultures and then started a combination of antibiotics active against all the bacteria I could think of. But clearing the bacteria out of Doris's blood would help only temporarily if I couldn't find out where the infection started. To cure Doris I would have to answer three questions: What germs are causing the infection? How did they get in? Where are they hiding now? I got a step stool so I could get up high enough to lean over Doris's bed and get my face in for a close look or a whiff of any wounds I might find. I lowered the bed rail and pulled on a pair of latex examination gloves. As I made these preparations I felt my confidence returning. This kind of medical detective work came naturally to me.

The first place I looked was the skin. Since Doris's immune system had been weakened by chemotherapy, bacteria could invade her blood stream even through a tiny break or a little infection. Her skin was sallow and clammy from shock and there were no areas of redness. I pulled off her socks and checked between each toe for the little cracks of athlete's foot. But there was nothing on the skin, not even a bug bite. I pulled her lower lids away from her eyes and looked for the red spots of endocarditis. Negative. I looked inside her eyes with an ophthalmoscope. No Roth spots. Alex and I rolled her over gently and checked her rectum for hemorrhoids and fissures. Nothing amiss down there.

I put my stethoscope against her chest, which was moving rapidly. Her lungs were full of coarse sounds, like fluid sloshing in the airways—pneumonia maybe, or the beginnings of shock lung. Her heart was normal, except that it was beating fast. I listened over her abdomen. There were rare gurgling sounds, so her intestines were still working. I felt Doris's liver on the right and then felt for her spleen on the left. Watching her face for a grimace of pain, I started at the top and I worked my way down to her belly, pushing hard. Doris's face remained impassive until I got to the lower left side. When I pushed there she winced slightly and opened her eyes.

"Does that hurt you, Doris?" I asked.

"A little, Doctor, like it did before," she answered in a whisper. Up to that moment, Doris had been a cool, moist object I was examining—a puzzle to solve. But when she winced under my hand and spoke, she became a person again.

I remembered that Doris had had a bout of colitis from her chemotherapy. She'd had blood-tinged diarrhea and inflammation of the large bowel. So her bowel was still tender. Could it be the source of her septic shock? An inflamed colon can be a portal to infection because the colon is normally filled with a whole metropolis of living bacteria separated from our insides by only the thin bowel wall.

Doris's oncologist, Dr. David O'Neill, came up to see his patient. We'd been residents together, and Dr. O'Neill, a tall, dignified fellow, had always been calm—he and I both practice meditation, but in his case, it seems to work. Oncologists focus on blood as well as on cancer, and Dr. O'Neill noted Doris's low platelet count and abnormal blood coagulation tests. He confirmed what I had feared. Doris had disseminated intravascular coagulation, or DIC, a condition in which the platelets and the clotting factors knit and unknit themselves in a septic frenzy, forming a clot and then dissolving it again. Dr. O'Neill was worried that the clotting system might become so depleted that Doris would bleed spontaneously. He recorded his assessment of her condition in her chart: "prognosis grave with high chance of demise."

That evening I was on call in the hospital. Before I went home at eight, I went back to the ICU to check on Doris. Her blood pressure was a little better, but on the second chest x-ray the normally black air-filled lungs now had the telltale white shadows of acute respiratory distress syndrome (ARDS). Bacterial toxins were unlocking the watertight seals in Doris's pulmonary blood vessels. Blood plasma was leaking into the air spaces so that oxygen wasn't being absorbed.

Of the complications of septic shock, ARDS seems among the hardest to treat once it gets under way. Any kind of shock can trigger it, even bleeding; in fact, the condition was previously called shock lung. But nowadays it most commonly occurs following serious infections. It doesn't matter if antibiotics kill all the bacteria in the patient's blood stream. In fact, some experts think that fragments of dead germs are just as toxic as the living ones.

Through the years, I've lost many patients to ARDS. When patients die of pneumococcal pneumonia, they usually die of ARDS. I see a case or two a year, usually in smokers over fifty with pneumonia and positive blood cultures. The pneumococcal vaccine could prevent some of these deaths, but antibiotics can't avert a fatal out-come once ARDS gets beyond the point of no return. Whatever the cause, every patient with ARDS is the same. The oxygen level in the blood falls and we dial up the oxygen in the ventilator tubing. But 100 percent oxygen is toxic to the lungs, so we try increasing the pressure at the end of each breath to drive the oxygen past the wet membranes into the blood stream. At this point, if the pa-tient's clinical condition improves, the lungs may gradually regain their integrity, stop leaking, and dry out. If not, the lungs eventually rupture from the pressure of each ventilator breath, or the oxygen level drops so low that the heart stops. On any given day in our ten-bed ICU there's usually at least one patient on a ventilator with ARDS. We keep them sedated so they won't fight the machine or try to yank the painful tubing out.

Doris had all the risk factors for ARDS. She was breathing 100 percent oxygen by facemask. I watched it steam up as she panted at a rate of thirty breaths a minute. She couldn't keep that up for long. I told the doctor to watch her carefully. If she tired, she would need to be put on the ventilator. Then I walked outside in the dark to my car, threw my white coat in the trunk, and drove home. It had been a long day.

When I came through the front door, my son, Paul, who was six then, threw his arms around me and kissed my cheek. He'd been waiting for me to read to him from *The Swiss Family Robinson*. Still in my work clothes, I pulled a chair up close to his bed and opened the book to where we had left off. The bedside lamp made a pool of light in the dark room. I started to read quietly about the father who was exploring an immense cave and "fired a pistol shot—the reverberating echoes of which testified to the great extent of the place." He lit a candle and advanced, "the light burning clear and steadily, though shedding a very feeble light in so vast a place."

Paul listened attentively from under the covers. His thick glasses lay on the bookshelf. He could not see me clearly without them because he had been born with cataracts and the lenses of his eyes had been removed in infancy. But he was looking up at the ceiling, seeing everything in his mind.

I watched him, and the events of my day receded.

The next day Doris's lungs failed. When I arrived at the ICU, the young pulmonary specialist, Dr. David Draper, was already talking to Sharon outside Doris's room. In a calm voice and in short clear sentences, he explained to her that it was time to attach her mother to a ventilator machine. She could no longer breathe on her own. I'd watched him have this talk with families before. He looked into Sharon's anxious face, his gaze kind and his manner decisive.

By two-thirty that afternoon, Doris was peacefully asleep on the ventilator, still under the influence of the drugs used to sedate her for the intubation procedure and exhausted by a night of hard breathing.

Later that same afternoon I got a call from our microbiology laboratory in North Hollywood. Doris's blood cultures were growing gram-negative rods, probably of intestinal origin. So there was a link, as I had suspected, between Doris's colon and her septic shock.

Sharon was sitting in Doris's room talking quietly to Alex, the nurse. He was patiently answering her questions about her mother's condition. A family member and the nurse taking care of a patient in the ICU spend hours together. I could see that these two had a good rapport, and I wondered how I would feel if it were my mother lying in that bed on a ventilator. I put my hand on Doris's shoulder and called her name. She opened her eyes but her gaze was unfocused. Her blood pressure was just out of shock range.

Doris's platelet count had dropped to thirty-four thousand, about one-quarter of the normal number. Still, she didn't have a fever and she was producing urine, both positive signs. Alex asked me to order a full liquid diet through a stomach tube for Doris, and Dr. Draper wanted to dial down the concentration of oxygen in the ventilator to avoid lung damage.

I wrote my note and went back to my office to start my morning clinic. The microbiology laboratory informed me that Doris's gram-negative rod was *Klebsiella*, a normal inhabitant of the human gut, but quite toxic in the blood stream.

When I returned to the ICU at five-thirty, I found Doris off dopamine and tolerating an oxygen concentration of only 40 percent—room air is 21 percent. Best of all, she seemed to recognize me and responded to my voice with a nod. She couldn't talk, of course, because of the plastic tube in her throat.

But Doris was not out of the woods yet. When I made my Saturday rounds the next day her platelet count had dropped further to twenty thousand, and at that level she could start bleeding at any time. I ordered platelet transfusions. Since she was on the right antibiotics for her *Klebsiella*, I wondered if I was missing something. Was some ICU bug invading her body? I removed all the intravenous and intra-arterial lines I could, hoping to minimize this risk. Dr. Draper thought her lungs were showing signs of improvement so, on that score, I felt encouraged.

That afternoon our family drove to Gardena, about thirty miles from our house, to attend a memorial service for my husband's grandfather, who had passed away thirty years earlier. With a cold coming on, I sniffled through the long Shinto ceremony, and when it was over, I was relieved to drowse in the back seat with my four-year-old daughter, Ellen. She was strapped into her car seat and eating a piece of soft candy. I could see her cloud of hair as she turned away to look out the window, the light shining through the whorl of her ear. Suddenly she started choking. Her face turned red and she gave me a terrible beseeching look. In a flash I unbuckled my seatbelt and lunged at her, clapping her between the shoulder blades. The candy came up. I wrapped my arms around her, tearful, my heart jumping in my throat. Then I sank back in my seat, listening to my pulse in my ears.

I woke up Sunday morning still miserable and made my hospital rounds in latex gloves, sniffling behind a paper mask. "Hi, Doris, how are you feeling?" I asked, although I knew she couldn't answer with the tube in. Doris was wide awake.

Dr. Draper came up the back stairs from the radiology department. "I think she's ready to come off the ventilator today," he said. "She's alert and her oxygen saturation is OK. We'll give her a trial of breathing on her own and then pull the tube if she does alright."

I went home and, after a quick nap, took Ellen to a birthday party on the posh south side of Ventura Boulevard in Encino. There were preschool classmates there that she talked about all the time, but they ignored her. She wasn't a part of their world of play dates because her mother worked and the other moms didn't. I sat on the grass, sad for Ellen. Then she came over and settled herself on my lap to watch Corey the clown. I put my arms around her and felt her chest move as she breathed. Suddenly perfectly happy, I nuzzled her hair.

When I made my rounds in the ICU on Monday, I found Doris off the ventilator, breathing a fifty-fifty mix of room air and humidified oxygen through a facemask. Doris had passed through the most perilous seven days of her life. She had survived the shock phase of her infection and also ARDS. I lifted the foggy mask partway off her face and asked, "How are you feeling, Doris?"

"I'm thirsty," she said in a hoarse voice.

"Well, welcome back. You've had quite a week," I said, putting the end of a flex straw in her mouth so she could drink cold water from a Styrofoam cup.

I listened to Doris's lungs and heart and then examined her abdomen. When I pressed down on the upper part of her belly, she grimaced.

"Does that hurt?" I asked, taking my hand away.

She nodded yes.

I noted Doris's abdominal tenderness in her chart, but I wasn't too concerned about it yet. Her belly was soft and the bowel sounds seemed normal. I was eager to get Doris's stomach tube out and to start feeding her. I ordered a trial of clear liquids. Doris was anemic from her ordeal so I gave her a two-unit blood transfusion.

Dr. Draper examined Doris very early on Tuesday. He wrote that she looked stronger but that she didn't recall any of the events of her past week in the hospital. When I examined her at nine, I was dismayed to find a measles-like rash over her trunk, a classic sign of drug allergy. I prescribed a different antibiotic and trans-ferred her out of the ICU.

Doris had made it out of intensive care, a minor miracle, but she was not safe yet. She'd had a fever of 102 during the night, and her white blood cell count was double what it should be. Still, her platelets were now normal, and I hoped that her fever was just part of her drug allergy.

In addition to Doris, I had a family matter to deal with. Ellen's nursery school ride arrangement had collapsed. My housekeeper didn't drive and I depended on other moms to bring Ellen home from preschool three days a week. I spent an anxious afternoon making phone calls between appointments.

The next day the physical therapists got Doris unsteadily to her feet for the first time. She said she was hungry, and I decided to try giving her a bland diet. I finished my morning clinic and went home to pick up Ellen. She was waiting with Gloria, our house-keeper, at the front door. When we got to the little adobe pre-school, I was so preoccupied with making sure her ride home was arranged that I left the school without pushing Ellen on the swing or saying goodbye. I was a mile away when I remembered. I turned the car around and headed back. Ellen was asking her teacher where I was and looking all over for me. I sat down on the play-ground steps with my daughter on my lap. Then she jumped up and kissed me goodbye, and I went back to work.

When I made rounds the next morning I could see that Doris had taken a turn for the worse. Her pulse was racing, she had a fever of over 101, and the right side of her belly was very tender. Her white blood cell count had climbed to three times normal. Was she going septic again, I wondered? I ordered an abdominal CT scan for the next day to find out the cause of Doris' abdominal tenderness and fever.

That night Paul came down with a temperature of 101 and threw up his supper. In the morning he looked better so I went to work. Doris had a temperature of almost 103. Then Gloria paged me. Paul had a high fever and was hallucinating. It was all I could do not to rush straight home, but I had a waiting room full of patients. I told Gloria to give Paul some more Tylenol and to sponge him off with tepid water. When I got home at 12:30 P.M. I rushed into the house.

"¿Cómo va el niño?" I asked Gloria. We went to Paul's room. He was sleeping peacefully in his clothes on top of his bed, his skin cool now.

Later that afternoon, Doris went down to the radiology department on the first floor for a CT scan of her abdomen. I was just finishing my clinic when the radiologist paged me.

"Your patient, Doris Silver, has a big low-density lesion in her liver."

"Big, like how big?" I asked. Low density meant liquid and liquid might mean pus.

"Big, like a baseball," he replied.

"Can you stick a needle in it? I think it might be an abscess."

"I can try."

I walked through radiology to the CT suite. The technician was seated at the computer console scrolling through Doris's computer-generated x-rays. The round white spot on her liver images was obvious, even to me. I walked past him into the shielded room containing the white ring of the CT scanner. Doris was lying on her left side on a narrow, wheeled table. The radiologist was putting a Band-Aid over the puncture he'd just made in her liver. He turned to the Mayo stand and handed me a syringe filled with thick beige pus. Pay dirt for an ID specialist.

As I walked down to the lab to make a Gram's stain of the specimen, I knew I had the key to Doris's illness in my hand. There under the microscope were a myriad of pink rods. So this was where the *Klebsiella* in her blood stream had come from. I guessed the germs had gone from her inflamed colon into the veins between the intestine and the liver. The liver normally filters out and destroys the few bacteria that find their way into the circulation. But, in Doris's case, either there were too many bacteria coming through at once, or her immune system was too weakened to filter the bacteria. The *Klebsiella* bacteria multiplied in the liver tissue and formed an abscess. When the abscess got large and the pressure inside it built up, bacteria were forced into the blood vessels draining the liver and got into the general circulation, producing septic shock.

Now I knew why Doris remained so ill despite all the antibiotics I'd been pouring into her. Antibiotics can only kill the bacteria in the blood stream. They can't cure an abscess, which has to be drained. The surgeons have a saying, "Where there's pus, let there be steel." And in the old days anyone with a liver abscess had to go under the knife in the operating room. But now with the CT scanner, the radiologist could drain the pus and bacteria using a little plastic tube.

I headed home. It was my tenth wedding anniversary, and the next day would be my first full day off in almost three weeks. That night Glenn and I celebrated peacefully, making different flavors of Jell-O for our children.

On Saturday, the radiologist inserted a drainage tube into Doris's abscess. She spent three more weeks in the hospital, but she eventually made a complete recovery. Her colon cancer never returned. Now I see her once or twice a year in my clinic for routine physical examinations and minor medical problems. She carries no physical trace of her terrible struggle ten years ago except some scarring at the base of her right lung where the plastic tube passed on its way to the liver.

Septic shock is one of the most common serious conditions doctors treat and it can affect any patient, from newborn babies to the elderly. About 45 percent of patients who develop the full-blown syndrome die, and patients who survive hang perilously between life and death, sometimes for days, while a team of health care professionals work around the clock to save them. Since time is critical in the treatment of septic shock, early recognition is essential. Fever, extreme weakness, and a drowsy confusion are the cardinal signs. But if the onset is insidious, as with Doris, or extremely rapid, the patient arrives at the hospital in the advanced stages. Then there is no escape, except through the shock syndrome and its complications and out the other side, either to life or to death.

Glenn and I still sit in the kitchen and drink decaf coffee. My work makes me introspective, and I asked him once after a hard week in the ICU, "What do you think is the meaning of life?"

My husband, who still likes to misunderstand me, answers, "I would have to say that the meanie of life would be Cruella De Vil or maybe Darth Vader."

He elaborates on this theme for a few minutes until, exasperated, I break in, "Not the meanie of life, dear. I asked you what was the mean*ing* of life?"

He thinks for a moment, then puts on a dour face and an Austrian accent and says, "To slay your enemies and to hear the lamentations of their women and children."

"That's your opinion?"

"No, but that's what Arnold Schwarzenegger says in *Conan the Barbarian*."

"Glenn, I really need to know what you think the meaning of life is!"

Seeing I'm not going to let him off the hook, he finally gives me his real opinion.

"The meaning of life is life itself. Life fighting to stay alive in a cold, dark universe."

And I have to agree.

The meaning of my life as a doctor is life itself and the struggle to keep it from flickering out under these annihilating attacks.

In the ICU, we are life's defenders. Every day we stand up for the patient against the cold and the dark that's waiting just beyond our ventilators, our antibiotics, and our stubborn ingenuity.

a case of chickenpox

He was a big, furry thing trapped under a traffic sawhorse at the bottom of my exit ramp. Every time he tried to get out, he was scared back by the rush of traffic. I pulled off, parked, and walked toward him—a short, middle-aged woman appearing out of the darkness wearing glasses and a white coat. "Get out of traffic, come on, let's go," I said. I was going to lead him to safety.

What happened is, I got drunk on being a savior and I started thinking I was supposed to save everything. The animal kingdom, too. I was on my way home that Friday night after a day in clinic plus a six-to-ten Urgent Care shift, and I'd seen so many patients, one after the other, that I was completely worn out. I had walked into those little exam rooms and solved each of their problems, and now I saw this dog as if it was the patient in room thirteen with a sore throat. I was in hospital mode—I'd forgotten that I wasn't there anymore.

I put out my hand to see if I could read his collar, and he started to lick my ragged cuticles. I reached for the collar again. The dog growled from a deep, primitive place, and lunged. Terrified, I backed away, then watched, as he seemed to forget me and his fear of the traffic, ambling off from under the sawhorse into the darkness. Only now I noticed that his gait was crooked and unsteady as he made his way down the street.

At that point, I realized I was an idiot. The dog looked sick, and I thought how stupid I'd been to let it lick me. Then I thought about how mad Glenn was going to be.

I walked back to my car and called up my ID colleague, Linda Croad. "Pam, it makes me nervous, and you sound nervous. Why don't you play it safe? Go to the ER and get some rabies immunoglobulin and vaccine."

By the end of the conversation I was home. My house is on a quiet street in Encino in what was once a walnut grove. I walked inside and headed straight to the sink. I took off my wedding ring and scrubbed my hands with antibacterial soap and bleach.

I poked my head into the children's rooms. Ellen and Paul were sleeping soundly. I went into our bedroom to tell Glenn what had happened.

He rolled his eyes and said, "Why did you do that?" He didn't wait for an answer. He reached for his pants and shoes. "I'll go and try to find it. What did it look like?"

"Look for Rin Tin Tin on marijuana," I said. "Like if Lassie and Rin Tin Tin were hippies and got together. What their puppies would look like."

"Well, at least you weren't bitten," Glenn said.

He returned twenty minutes later having had no luck. I drove myself back to the hospital and sat in the emergency room with other patients, waiting to see the doctor. When I did see him, I was matter-of-fact: "I got licked by a stray dog that was acting bizarrely."

The doc filled out a dog-bite form and gave me a shot in the butt of rabies immunoglobulin. The substance works like a vacuum cleaner, sucking up any virus particles loose in the blood stream. In my left arm I got my first shot of the bright red rabies vaccine. It's made from human cells grown in tissue culture (instead of duck embryo cells like the earlier vaccines), and unlike the old rabies shots, doesn't have to be given into the abdominal muscles, though it still hurts. My series of rabies vaccines would consist of additional shots on days 3, 7, 14, and 28. All I could think of as I left the ER was, "You've got to stop trying to rescue everything."

That night I dreamed a woodsman came down from a mountain. A big wooden cart followed him. At each point on the cart where a wheel should have been, was a dog. But on the right front axle, the dog was missing. After a moment, the dog from the freeway exit ramp loped up and filled the space. With a great shout, the woodsman and the cart wound past me and then disappeared into the distance.

My clinic was so busy that over the following weeks I wound up ducking into the copy room and giving myself those bright red injections. But that dog was just the latest in a series of my mad rescues. Like that guy in 1994, I thought ruefully as I took off my white coat and rolled up my sleeve, like Charlie.

It was a Friday afternoon when the paramedics brought him in. It was a terrible case. The man's own mother would not have recognized him. His entire face was swollen and bloody, and his shoulders were raw, like a burn victim. Mixed in with the blood was yellow pus that filled the exam room with the smell of decay. On his trunk, black ulcers were surrounded by normal skin, but on his face, there was no intact skin at all. His gray-blue eyes peered at me from under swollen lids with mute appeal. Shocked and nauseated, I wondered what infectious disease had done this.

I asked the paramedics for their report.

"Charlie Blair, a forty-year-old male, BP 84/62, pulse 120, temp 99.2. Diagnosis: chickenpox."

A virus of the herpes family called VZV causes chickenpox, or varicella. The herpes viruses are among the giants of the virus world, but they're still less than one-fourth the size of a bacterium. A miserable, but usually self-limited disease in childhood, varicella can be life threatening in adults.

Charlie was in early shock. I could see the pus on his ulcerated skin, and I suspected his chickenpox lesions had become infected with bacteria, which were now invading his blood stream. He was dehydrated, but he was also septic.

I pushed my horror to one side and got down to work. Leaning over closely to a particularly soupy area, I took a thoughtful sniff. "Musty," I said to myself. "Maybe staph." The odor of an organism can be as identifying as a fingerprint. The pus in a Pseudomonas infection may smell yeasty or fruity. It may be bluish green, too. If a diabetic's infected foot smells like stool, I think of bacteria that live without oxygen. Charlie smelled musty, mousy, like *Staphylococcus aureus*. If that bug had gotten into his blood, he was in big trouble. Charlie's skin was no longer protecting him, and he had become fertile ground for multiplying microorganisms.

Two young men and a young woman were standing anxiously at Charlie's bedside. One man was his roommate and the other two people were friends from work. "Charlie's been sick for a week," said the woman, "It started last Friday, and by Sunday the rash was so bad we took him to an ER. Since he doesn't have any medical insurance, they sent him downtown to a county hospital."

"How long did they keep him there?" I asked.

"He came home two days later, on Tuesday morning," she answered. "They said he had some hepatitis from chickenpox, but they thought he was getting better."

"Did they give him any pills to take?" I asked, wondering if he'd been given the antiviral drug acyclovir.

"No," she answered. "After we brought him home, the rash spread all over his face and down the back of his neck. He had fevers every night."

"But yesterday he started to look better," interrupted one of the men.

"He walked around the apartment and we gave him some soup," said the other.

The young woman resumed her story. "Then early this morning, we found him talking crazy. He seemed upset. When we tried to stand him up, he fainted. That was it. I called 911 and we followed the ambulance here." She leaned toward me. "Do you think he's going to be OK?"

"We'll do our best," I said, but I was puzzled. If I'd had an adult patient sick enough with chickenpox to be admitted to the hospital, I'd have given him acyclovir and I wouldn't have sent him out so fast. Well, it was a good thing they had found me, an ID expert, I thought. I knew what I was doing and, as sick as this patient was, I felt confident I could save him.

According to his friends, Charlie had been a healthy, athletic person, though they had only known him about a year. He had moved out to California to be closer to his sons, aged eleven and thirteen, who lived with their mother in Anaheim. The boys had been visiting him a week before he got sick. Toward the end of the visit, the youngest came down with chickenpox.

Charlie wasn't a member of our HMO, but he was too unstable to be transferred anywhere.

"I'm going to admit Charlie to the hospital. I want you three to go home now and get some rest." I ordered samples of his blood to be drawn for cultures and other tests. Charlie had lost perhaps a quarter of his body fluid because of his fever and skin wounds, from which water was continuing to evaporate at an enormous rate. To further complicate matters, he had not been able to eat or drink much. "Run in normal saline with the IV wide open," I told the ER nurse.

Next, I called the in-patient pharmacy. "Chuck, I've got a guy in the ER with bacterial sepsis on top of chickenpox. Would you bring up a gram of Vanco and two grams of Ceftizox, STAT?" I gave him Charlie's name and approximate weight. "And Chuck, he's very dry. His creatinine's 2.9, so we'll have to dose him carefully." A normal creatinine is 1.0, and Charlie's kidneys were showing the effects of dehydration. In addition to the antibiotics, I also started Charlie on an intravenous drip of acyclovir. Unlike antibiotics, which actually kill bacteria, antiviral medicines can only inhibit viruses. If Charlie were to recover, his immune system would have to inactivate the varicella virus on its own. I was hoping the acyclovir would help him in his struggle.

I dictated a history and physical, wrote orders for the care of his wounds, and, as varicella is a very contagious disease by air, arranged for a bed in an isolation room for Charlie on the medical ward. Only nurses who had a positive blood test for past chickenpox infection in their employee files would be assigned to take care of him.

"His chest x-ray's still clear," I told his friends as they were leaving, "and that's a good sign."

Charlie seemed to be resting comfortably when I checked on him that evening. It was Friday, and I was looking forward to a weekend off.

When I returned to work on Monday, Charlie was sitting up in bed with his breakfast tray in front of him. He had a pale green oxygen tube in his nose, and his voice was a little hoarse. "How do you feel?" I asked.

He smiled weakly with bloody lips and said, "Better." His chart showed he had only a little fever. His blood pressure was normal but his pulse was ninety. I looked under the plastic cover over the plate on his breakfast tray. Charlie had not eaten anything. There was something else, more worrisome still: He was breathing thirty-two times a minute (the normal rate is less than twenty times a minute).

Because of Charlie's wounds, I put on latex gloves before I examined him. I've had chickenpox, so I didn't bother with a mask. As I moved my stethoscope over his chest, I heard the normal to-and-fro sound of air moving through his lungs. The crackles of pneumonia are more like two pieces of Velcro being pulled apart. Then I felt his abdomen. It was tense and slightly distended. I pressed more deeply. "Does that hurt?" I asked, watching Charlie's face. "No," he said, and his expression did not change.

My stethoscope was soiled with blood and pus from Charlie's wounds. I disinfected it with soap, water, and alcohol and sat down at the nurse's station with his chart. His creatinine was 2.7, but his platelet count was now almost in the normal range. Taken together with his blood pressure, the normal platelet count suggested that his septic state was clearing with antibiotic treatment.

I went down to the x-ray department on the first floor. The x-rays taken that day and the previous one were posted on the alternator, a long rotating machine with numbered banks of lighted boxes. I looked up the number of Charlie's film from the list and pushed the foot pedal to start the alternator moving. Charlie's x-ray swung into view. On the left was the chest x-ray taken in the ER, and next to it was the film of that morning. There was an ominous haziness at the base of the left lung, near the heart, which had not been visible the previous day. Charlie had been so dehydrated when he came in that he could have had that pneumonia all along and I would not have seen it on the first film. The intravenous fluids we gave him flooded the inflamed lung and made the abnormality visible. "I bet this pneumonia is what made him go off his rocker the night before he came in," I thought.

My nose instincts were right about the bacteria on Charlie's skin. The blood cultures started turning positive over the weekend, and by Monday, all four bottles were growing *Staphylococcus aureus*. A small round bacterium that grows in clusters, *Staphylococcus aureus* looks like a bunch of grapes, *staphyle* in Greek. When grown in agar plates, the organism produces orange-yellow pigment, so the colonies may appear golden, *aureus*. Staph has been infecting people since prehistoric times. It causes most of the skin abscesses that require surgical drainage. The bacterium is equipped with a whole battery of enzymes and toxins. It is quite capable of invading the blood stream, as in Charlie's case, and causing septic shock. But was staph the cause of Charlie's pneumonia, or was it varicella? I would have to assume that both were playing a role.

On my rounds the next morning, I found Charlie on the high-acuity ward. He had had some breathing problems during the night and had been moved for closer observation. When I asked, Charlie said his breathing was "better." The chickenpox lesions were the same. He had eaten some breakfast and his wheezes were gone. "Cough, Charlie," I said. He made a wet cough, which worried me. There was plenty of stuff in his lungs.

He was definitely stoical. I was sure he was minimizing his symptoms. There is an instinct, especially among people with physical courage, to hide their suffering, like a wounded animal trying to keep up with the herd. Charlie kept saying that he was feeling "better," but was he really? He didn't even seem to be hearing me very well.

I thought the drugs might be making him deaf, so I got an otoscope from the supply room and looked in his ears. Each ear canal was tightly plugged by a maroon blood clot. The chickenpox lesions in his ears had filled them with fresh blood! I shook my head with amazement.

On the high-acuity ward, Charlie was being cared for by an excellent registered nurse named Frank. He had been a medic with the Army Special Forces in Vietnam (the Green Berets), returned safely home, and was married with two children. "I think the other nurses were afraid to take care of Charlie," he told me later. "He looked creepy, like the old newsreels of smallpox. All of a sudden, they weren't so sure they'd had the chickenpox." Frank gently cleaned out Charlie's ears.

The next day Charlie's shortness of breath was much worse, but his lungs still sounded pretty clear with the stethoscope. Puzzled, I ordered another chest x-ray. His pneumonia was perhaps a little worse, but there was a second, completely unexpected, finding. Underneath both sides of the diaphragm, which separates the chest from the abdominal cavity, was a bubble of free air. Since there are no air bubbles in the abdominal cavity, this could only mean one thing. Charlie had a perforation, a hole, somewhere in his intestinal system. There was nothing I could do about this problem with medicine. The hole would have to be closed in the operating room as soon as possible or peritonitis would set in. (Similar to a ruptured appendix, if bacteria leak out of any hole in the intestine, they cause a raging infection inside the abdominal cavity.)

At noon that day, Dr. Steven Stein, the same surgeon who had operated on the strep patient, Allan Roth, came to see Charlie. Dr. Stein, then in his thirties, is of medium height, with dark brown hair and a neat beard. He's very incisive and has a talent for being right about things. He found Charlie's abdomen to be distended, but still soft. The boardlike rigidity of peritonitis had not yet set in. He wrote in the chart: "free intraperitoneal air, disseminated varicella. Patient most likely with intestinal perforation due to viral involvement of the intestine." Charlie's chickenpox was not confined to his skin; it had spread (disseminated) to involve many of his internal organs as well. In this most dangerous form of the disease, the multiplying varicella virus explodes the host's cells causing spots of dead tissue. If one of these spots was in the gastrointestinal tract, it would leak air and fluid.

That afternoon, Charlie went to the OR, where Dr. Stein repaired a quarter-inch hole in his stomach where a chickenpox lesion had eaten through the wall. During this surgery, Dr. Stein had the rare opportunity to observe severe chickenpox inside a living patient. In his operative report he noted the cause of Charlie's abnormal liver tests: "firm liver with petechiae/hemorrhage compatible with varicella hepatitis." The liver itself was dotted with chickenpox lesions.

The next day, Charlie was breathing more normally. Even though I now had a patient with a big, midline surgical incision, I tried to convince myself he would be eating soon. I resumed the treatment of his skin with wet to dry dressings and Silvadene ointment. Like a burn victim, Charlie had lost most of the outer layer of his skin so I was giving him the same kind of treatment burn patients receive.

Charlie began to unravel the following day. The anesthesiologist was paged STAT to the high-acuity ward. Charlie was gasping for breath and his oxygen level was dropping. The anesthesiologist passed a plastic tube from Charlie's mouth, through his trachea, and into his lungs to give him oxygen. It was not an easy intubation because there was swelling just below the larynx. When the pulmonary specialist examined Charlie's airway, he saw that the swelling was caused by chickenpox lesions that were making the lining of his trachea slough off, just like in his ear canals. The debris and swelling had obstructed Charlie's breathing passage, choking him.

Charlie was now in the intensive care unit, intubated and dependent on a ventilator. He was the focus of an intense team effort. What had started as my case in the emergency room now became the concern of over a dozen doctors, nurses, pharmacists, and respiratory therapists. Almost everyone working in our hospital knew about the struggle that was going on in the ICU.

Dr. Elsa Bergman, the family practice resident working on the renal service with her attendings, left daily instructions on how much and what kinds of fluids to give my patient to support his kidneys. The pulmonary specialists, Doctors Draper, Ng, and Robyns, were struggling to minimize the damage to Charlie's lungs, for it was clear now that he had chickenpox lesions there as well. The surgeon, Steven Stein, was attending to Charlie's abdominal wound. The ICU nurses were spending long shifts with Charlie, who, while trapped on the ventilator and unable to talk, was communicating by gestures and by writing words on a clipboard. Frank, his nurse from high acuity, was now taking care of him in the ICU.

At about this time, Charlie's ex-wife, Joanne, began to bring their eleven and thirteen-year-old sons to visit him. Joanne is an RN and lives in Anaheim, about sixty miles from the hospital. She had not been able to come earlier because she had been caring for their eldest son, who had come down with severe chickenpox as his brother was getting over it. Now they were reluctant to touch him. Even his hands were rough and strange. However, on the end of Charlie's right index finger was the soft, red light of his pulse-oximeter, monitoring the oxygen content of his blood. Charlie would hold up his hand and touch fingers with his sons, like in the movie *E.T.*

On May 8, two days after Charlie went into respiratory failure, my pharmacists reported that the *Staphylococcus aureus* in Charlie's sputum had been replaced by a new, more drug-resistant micro-organism, *Pseudomonas aeruginosa,* the same hospital organism that had melted Allan Roth's skin graft. The lungs of a patient on a ventilator become a breeding place for resistant germs that find their way down the endotracheal tube, and may even colonize the water mist used to moisten the patient's oxygen. The longer the patient is on the ventilator, the worse the situation gets. I added two new antibiotics to Charlie's regimen, and stopped one that wasn't working any more, but I was running out of options. It was as if the varicella and staph had been the predators, and now Pseudomonas was coming in like a scavenger to feed on my defenseless patient.

Despite all this, I didn't lose hope. In my note the next day, I wrote that Charlie was "awake, alert, and in good spirits." However, he had a temperature of almost 100 and yellow secretions poured from his endotracheal tube. Charlie's blood count was 26 percent (normal is 42), so I gave him a transfusion of two units of blood.

May 10 was day eleven in the hospital. In addition to Pseudomonas, Charlie's sputum started growing a mold called Aspergillus. Aspergillus is a fungus, similar to the ones that grow on bread. It does not cause disease in normal people. It was another scavenger feeding on my patient's damaged lungs. Charlie's blood oxygen level was low, and he now had pneumonia in his left lung as well as in his right. I began itraconazole, an antifungal drug.

Later that afternoon, Charlie's endotracheal tube became dislodged and had to be removed. Dr. Brian Ng, a neat man in his mid-thirties, decided to observe Charlie off the ventilator to see if he could breathe on his own. The next day when I made my rounds, Charlie was still off the ventilator, although he required 100 percent oxygen through a facemask. I was elated and decided to take the latex catheter out of Charlie's bladder. I wrote a note in the chart about feeding him and about simplifying his antibiotics. Dr. Ng wrote that Charlie was "without any complaints of shortness of breath." Ever stoical, Charlie was actually breathing at the exhausting rate of thirty times a minute. The resident on pulmonary medicine, rounding an hour after me, noticed that Charlie was "working slightly more today with breathing," and that his chest x-ray looked a little worse.

The next morning I was upset to find Charlie back on the ventilator. At 2 A.M. his blood oxygen had fallen to dangerous levels and the tube had to be put back in. He had a fever of 101.4 and a pulse of 128. He was severely anemic again and needed more blood. His chest x-ray showed the most serious pulmonary abnormality, acute respiratory distress syndrome, or ARDS. The lung tissue had lost its watertight seal and become soggy, and it couldn't absorb gases, even with 100 percent oxygen on a ventilator. That morning, Dr. Ng wrote one of his long logical notes. His assessment: "the inflammatory/capillary leak process appears to be overwhelming."

Doctors make use of denial, just as patients do. It's one of the ways we cling to our savior fantasies, long after the saving part of patient care is over. None of us talked explicitly about Charlie's condition. We didn't want to admit, even to ourselves, that he might not make it. Locked in a struggle like this one, the only way to function is to focus on details, at the expense of the big picture, and to go on one day at a time. Even the RN, Frank, fell under the spell of his hopes.

He tried a special form of inhaled epinephrine in the ventilator tubing and was so encouraged by the initial clearing of Charlie's secretions that he said, "In my own naive way, I thought we had turned the corner."

Whole books have been written about how important it is for patients not to lose hope. But hope is important to doctors and nurses as well. There can't be any confidence without it. But, while hope can create strength, it's a double-edged sword. In order to feel hope you have to let your emotional guard down and be vulnerable, and you have to close your eyes to certain facts. But while the experienced among us always know what's going on to some degree, the young residents may not. We were horrified when a young doctor quipped to Charlie's sons, "Which one of you boys gave your dad the chickenpox?" But it was really our fault for not being clear, to ourselves and to him.

Charlie's skin began to heal, but the liver damage from the varicella worsened. His eyes became so bright with jaundice that his frightened sons thought they were actually glowing with yellow light.

Despite his condition, Charlie was upbeat and alert. He continued to write notes on his clipboard. He told Frank that he would tolerate anything we did to him in the ICU, if only he could have a Diet Coke. When Charlie was frightened, his pulse and blood pressure would go up. Then Frank would speak to him gently and tell him to breathe quietly. The medic who held the hands of dying soldiers in Vietnam now held Charlie's.

Charlie developed more complications. A nasogastric tube perforated his already damaged left lung, and a chest tube had to be inserted into the left chest cavity to keep his lung from collapsing.

Charlie's sister flew in from Louisiana. Dr. Ng noted in Charlie's chart: "multi-organ system failure, ARDS, the fact that the pulmonary infiltrates progressed this week is not a good prognostic sign." In other words, Charlie's x-rays were worsening. Instead of dark spaces in the lung where air was supposed to be, the films were becoming progressively whiter as fluid, pus, and scar tissue blocked the path of the x-rays to the film.

By the second week in May, Charlie was as sick with the complications of ICU treatment as he was from varicella. We were fighting a battle on many fronts. To the original virus were now added bacterial and fungal invaders of his damaged lungs. He had surgical wounds in his abdomen and chest cavity that weren't healing because of his poor general condition. And Charlie's plastic endotracheal tube, which passed from his mouth between his vocal cords and into his windpipe, had been in place for twelve days. It could not stay in much longer.

On May 19, I sat down to talk to Dr. D. B. Robyns, the pulmonary specialist on call in the ICU that week. Dr. Robyns, then fifty, is an ex-air force officer with thick black hair and moustache, a clear thinker who can weigh all the alternatives dispassionately. We knew that it was time to talk to Charlie about a tracheotomy, which would allow us to connect the ventilator directly to his windpipe so that he could be kept on the breathing machine for months, even for life, if necessary.

That morning I noted that Charlie was "awake, alert, cheerful," and I thought that he was breathing better. Dr. Robyns pointed out that despite the damage to his lungs, Charlie was making some progress with "weaning off the ventilator." The latest measurements he had taken showed that Charlie had a fair chance of breathing on his own without the machine. In addition, if he could avoid the tracheotomy, he wouldn't have to breathe against the resistance of a plastic tube and he would be able to speak.

We went to the bedside to explain the situation to Charlie, who looked up at us calm and alert. Although a dense helmet of scab still covered his head, Charlie's face was almost healed now and was not scarred. He was being restored, at least on the outside, and seemed like a prince escaping an enchantment. Charlie was a handsome man with a broad brow, a fine straight nose, and large gray-blue eyes.

In simple terms we explained his options to him. Was he willing to try taking the tube out? He nodded yes.

On May 20, the tube was removed from Charlie's trachea. On the next day he had his first normal meal since before his surgery. I ordered emollients for his scalp to start to remove his "blood helmet" without pulling out his hair.

The next day Charlie coughed up a little blood and became temporarily short of breath. His oxygen saturation dropped. His sputum was now growing an organism that was resistant to seven different antibiotics.

Charlie's ex-wife came with the boys. Because of swelling around his vocal cords from the tube, he still hadn't regained his voice. At the end of the visit, he looked up at her and mouthed the words, "Thank you."

"It was as if he was saying goodbye," she said.

By the fourth day it was clear that Charlie was not going to be able to breathe without the ventilator. He was panting, and I could feel his heart pounding underneath my stethoscope. During the night he had coughed up more blood; now he was having trouble forcing the air out of his lungs. I wrote, "doing poorly today." Later that morning the plastic tube had to be replaced, and he was hooked back up on the machine.

That night Charlie became confused and agitated. The nurses tied his wrists to the bed rails but somehow he managed to grab the tubing connecting him to the ventilator. He pulled the endotracheal tube out of his mouth, his heart stopped beating, and the doctors could not resuscitate him. The next day when I came to the ICU he was gone.

Charlie had been the focus of everyone's attention for almost a month and we mourned him. Frank still remembers him vividly, and if you ask any nurse who cared for him in the ICU, even years later, they will point out his room. Everyone remembers the man who died of chickenpox.

In March 1995, a year after Charlie died, a live varicella vaccine was licensed in the United States. The virus in the vaccine is weakened in the laboratory, so that it produces only a mild infection, usually without symptoms. Afterward the patient has long-lasting immunity to the disease. Varicella vaccine is now widely used in children and is quite safe. But the vaccine is also very useful and important in adults who have not had the disease. Every year in the United States, young adults like Charlie die of chickenpox. In May 1997, the Centers for Disease Control and Prevention in Atlanta reported the deaths of three young women from chickenpox. All three of these deaths might have been prevented by varicella vaccine.

Research has shown that when people say they've had chickenpox, they're usually immune to the disease. When a person is unsure or thinks he may not have had chickenpox, a simple blood test can identify those who are susceptible and who should be vaccinated.

People still think of chickenpox as an uncomfortable but benign disease, but in Charlie's case, the varicella virus caused an invasive, widespread infection with irreversible damage by the time he was brought to us. He came to our hospital in trouble, and like Good Samaritans we embraced his care. Determined to save him, we refused to believe, even up to the end, that we were going to lose a young man to chickenpox. We never gave up hope.

chapter 11

call me spot

The kids and I had just returned from a pool party in Thousand
Oaks where we were treated to an abundance of low-fat food that
tasted awful. I was rummaging through our refrigerator looking for
something decent to eat when my beeper went off.

It was Thai Nguyen in Urgent Care. "Pam, I've got a kid here
who looks pretty sick. He has a high fever and his pulse is 130. He's
got weird purple skin lesions that look like hemorrhages. Some are
running together. Do you think it's an infected heart valve? His
name is Jeremy Albright. He's twenty."

I had an immediate image of Jeremy as an eight-year-old. His
mother, Alice, was an RN, and Jeremy had volunteered to be a medical model for an advanced cardiac life support class. He had worn
swimming trunks as we marked up his body with red, blue, and
green ink to show veins, arteries, and bones. A bright, enthusiastic
boy, he knew what he wanted to be when he grew up: president of
the United States.

I sat down on a kitchen chair and thought about that purple rash. "It might be something a lot worse. It might be meningococcal sepsis. Do a lumbar puncture. I'm on my way."

Nowadays we hear a lot about the viral hemorrhagic fevers in Africa, like Ebola, which is fatal in up to 80 percent of cases; it's a real "slate wiper." But a bacterium, the meningococcus, can cause hemorrhagic fever, too, and you don't have to go to Africa to catch it.

To begin with, the meningococcus, or *Neisseria meningitidis,* is not rare. Human beings are its only known host (it lives in the back of our throats), and we frequently entertain it without harm. Microscopically, it looks quite innocuous, practically charming. When Gram-stained, it appears pink and resembles a pair of kissing kidney beans. It travels from person to person by air. Almost everyone reading this sentence has been a carrier of the meningococcus, at one time or another, probably for months. The bug is stealthy. It mostly lives with us, but once in a while, some invisible balance tilts in its direction; it goes berserk and kills everyone in the house.

No one is exactly sure what changes the meningococcus from a harmless commensal to a deadly invader. The risk is highest when people first become carriers, probably because new carriers lack protective antibodies to the germ. Carrying the organism in the throat acts as a natural immunizer; the body learns to recognize the meningococcus and make protective antibodies against it. Patients get sick if these and other defenses fail and the bacterium escapes the membranes of the throat, enters the blood stream, and multiplies unchecked.

The telltale rash covering Jeremy's body was first described in 1806 in a village near Geneva. A physician named Gaspard Vieusseux reported an outbreak of something he called "malignant purpuric fever." The illness "began in a most peculiar and terrifying manner at a very small distance from the town, in a district inhabited by poor people . . . At the end of January, in a family composed of a woman and three children, two of the children were attacked and died in less than forty-eight hours." Fifteen days later, four of five children in a nearby family died of the disease. He continued, "a young man living in a house nearby was also attacked by the same disease and died between evening and morning, having a purple body, even to the tips of his fingers." This rash gave the most aggressive form of meningococcal disease its name, *purpura fulminans. Purpura,* Latin for purple; *fulminans,* from *fulminare,* to be struck by lightning.

When I arrived at the clinic twenty minutes later, three doctors were gently rolling Jeremy onto his side for a spinal tap. His face wrinkled into a grimace each time he was touched or moved. It was terrible to see him in such pain.

When he saw me, Jeremy smiled weakly and said, "Hi, Pam. I feel awful."

"I know, Jeremy," I said, "but you're going to be OK."

He had grown tall, lean, and handsome. His blond hair was the same as when he was a kid.

Alice and her husband, John, were in the waiting room. I took Alice aside. She is a short rotund woman, alert, ordinarily unflappable, a typical ER nurse. Tonight she was restless and looked terrified.

"What happened?" I asked.

"Last night, Jeremy said he felt really tired. He went to bed early. He woke up at 5:30 this morning with a fever of 101 and terrible back pain. At first he seemed to be doing all right, drinking fluids, resting in bed. Then at 2:30 this afternoon, I saw a rash on the back of his left hand. By then his temperature was 103. I knew those little bleeding spots under the skin were serious. As I watched him over the next half hour, more and more of them appeared. I thought, 'Oh Lord, could he have leukemia?' I told John and Jeremy, 'We're going to the hospital right now!'"

Alice stared at me, intently focused on what I would say next. I hugged her and said, "Listen, it's great you got him here so fast. I think it's meningococcemia. We're going to take good care of him."

Alice nodded and squeezed my hand. I watched her return to her place next to John. I couldn't bring myself to tell them that there was maybe a 40 percent chance that Jeremy wouldn't make it.

As I put a paper mask over my nose and mouth, my mind was gauging the risk of contracting a life-threatening disease. With someone like Jeremy, who has something really virulent, I knew the risk was significant. *Neisseria meningitidis* is contagious from person to person by the respiratory route. Carriers and patients sick with the disease exhale the organism into the air around them in the form of tiny infectious droplets. But a simple paper mask is fairly protective.

I walked into the room to examine my patient. Robert, the intern in family practice who was working with me that month, was waiting at the bedside, a paper mask already covering his mouth and nose. Dr. Nguyen and another resident, also in masks, were setting up the instrument tray for the spinal tap. We tried not to get too close to Jeremy's face. None of us wanted to take this germ home to our families.

The inside of Jeremy's left lower eyelid turned bright red as we watched. The blood-red spots under his skin were enlarging visibly as we examined him. I put my gloved hand gently on his arm and said, "How are you doing, Jeremy?"

"Awful," was all he said, his eyes bright with fear. He looked like a hunted animal. I recognized his fright as another symptom of septic shock. Septic patients often have a terrible sense of impending doom.

"We're going to take care of you, Jeremy. You hang in there, OK?" His pulse was racing at 120 beats a minute and his blood pressure was dropping. I wrote in his chart, "scattered petechiae of all sizes, largest one is pustular [pimple-like] on left index finger and exquisitely painful. Entire body is tender to touch."

I didn't want to watch the resident slip the long spinal needle into Jeremy's lower back. My intern and I left the room. We sat down in an adjoining examination room.

"Robert, I've known this kid since he was a little boy, and this is a real difficult one for me. I'm losing it here."

I was so anxious, so grieved that I could hardly think. I tried to maintain control the way doctors always do, by talking about the disease instead of the patient.

"What else besides meningococcal sepsis is in the differential diagnosis of a petechial rash in a patient with high fever?"

"Streptococcal sepsis and staphylococcal sepsis," Robert replied, sitting up straighter because he was being questioned by his attending.

"Yes," I said, "and we'll have to cover those. What else?"

"Infectious endocarditis," he answered.

"That's right, an infected heart valve throwing showers of little clots off the valve. Anything else?" He hesitated. I helped him, "Viral hemorrhagic fevers, like Ebola and Marburg, neither of which occur in California, and one other illness that occasionally does, Rocky Mountain spotted fever. We'll have to cover that one, too. We'll definitely have to shotgun him—cover everything."

There was really no time to waste. Antibiotics had to be started immediately. Having reviewed the possibilities, I was more convinced than ever that Jeremy was suffering from meningococcemia. I was haunted by something I had read about the infection: "The capacity of the meningococcus to kill a perfectly healthy individual within a few hours remains one of the most awesome characteristics of this disease." I left the room to find Jeremy's parents.

"Does Jeremy have any allergies to antibiotics?"

"Yes," said Alice. "When he was three years old he was given penicillin for an ear infection and got real bad hives."

I shook my head and sat down. This really wasn't turning out to be my day. "Hives can be a sign of a serious allergy. I can't risk giving Jeremy a related drug. He could have breathing problems or go into shock." Then, turning to Alice, I said, "I'm going to have to give him chloramphenicol."

Chloramphenicol is a drug that has a bad name among doctors and nurses in the United States. Not long after it was released in 1949, cases of aplastic anemia began to appear in people who had received it by mouth or injection. In aplastic anemia, patients' bone marrow, the place where blood cells are made, is damaged. In the chloramphenicol cases, the aplastic anemia often began weeks or even months after the patients had recovered from the infection for which they had been treated. They came to the hospital pale, with bleeding or infection. All of the patients who came down with aplastic anemia from taking the drug died.

Aplastic anemia following chloramphenicol administration was and is very rare. It only occurs in one in twenty-four to forty-eight thousand people receiving the antibiotic. Since the drug is cheap and effective, it is still used extensively in the Third World to treat infections. But in the United States, where alternatives are almost always available, no physician is willing to risk giving his or her patient a fatal disease. So the drug is rarely used except in patients with suspected meningococcal disease or Rocky Mountain spotted fever who have dangerous allergies to penicillin.

Alice knew about chloramphenicol as well as I did, but she had confidence in me. She told me to go ahead. I felt the familiar weight of responsibility descend on my shoulders, and with it, the implications of her trust. She had put her son's life in my hands.

I telephoned the pharmacy. Yes, they had some chloramphenicol. "Good," I said. "Put a gram of it in an IV piggyback and run it up here, STAT."

Jeremy's situation was so critical that as soon as the resident caught the first drops of cerebrospinal fluid in the plastic collection tube, I hung the chloramphenicol myself instead of waiting for a nurse to do it. I also ordered two other non-penicillin antibiotics to cover the remaining diseases Robert and I had discussed. Then I left Robert in charge. He was scheduled to spend the night in the hospital and would keep a watchful eye on Jeremy. We both knew that our patient would either start to get better, or begin a fatal downhill slide over the next few hours. We had done everything we could for now.

I spent an anxious night and headed for the intensive care unit first thing the next morning. I overcame my impulse to go straight to Jeremy's corner isolation room. Forcing myself to look methodically through his chart, I saw that his lumbar puncture was negative for meningitis, which was a relief to me. The vital signs sheet showed that his fever had disappeared, only to be replaced by a more disturbing sign, a subnormal temperature. His blood pressure had been under 100 systolic all night (normal is 120), so he was still in septic shock.

I put Jeremy's chart down and went over to his room. There was a respiratory isolation sign on the closed door and a box of disposable masks on the railing. I put one on and went in. Jeremy was hooked up to the cardiac monitor. His pulse was between ninety and one hundred. He was wearing oxygen and an IV was infusing antibiotics and fluid into an arm vein.

"How are you feeling?" I asked.

"Much better," he said, without sitting up. Jeremy's rash covered even more of his body than it had the day before and was absolutely classic for meningococcemia.

"Call me Spot!" he said, smiling crookedly from where he lay in bed.

I went to the computer and punched up Jeremy's laboratory tests for that morning. His white blood count had risen to almost twenty-five thousand, which was actually a good sign. In meningococcal sepsis, if the body can't mount a high white count, it means that the immune defenses are still not doing their job. His platelets, however, were low, and tests showed that his infection was setting off a chain reaction in his blood stream. The clotting factors in his blood were being destroyed, causing more bleeding within his rash. On the other hand, Jeremy's kidney function, which had been impaired on admission, was now back to normal, a very good sign. Jeremy was holding his own.

Jeremy's blood cultures were not growing anything yet. That could take several days. I knew I couldn't wait that long to inform the public health department about Jeremy. As long as he was kept in isolation and we were careful about wearing masks, we were relatively safe from Jeremy's infection. But what about the people who had been in close contact with him in the two or three days before his admission to the hospital?

The CDC includes *Neisseria meningiditis* on the list it publishes of "Clinical Syndromes Warranting Additional Empiric Precautions to Prevent Transmission . . . Pending Confirmation of Diagnosis." In other words, a disease on this list is an infectious disease emergency. Invasive meningococcal disease can spread quickly to people in close contact with a patient. The attack rate for those who live in the same house with a patient like Jeremy has been estimated to be four cases per one thousand persons exposed, which is five to eight hundred times greater than for the population at large. People exposed outside the home can also be affected. In a February 1991 outbreak in a classroom in Texas, five classmates and two siblings of an ill child came down with meningococcal disease and one died. Classmates whose seats were less than 100 centimeters "nose to nose" from the first cases were at greatest risk. In 1993, eight inmates of the Los Angeles County Jail fell ill with the disease. Before the epidemic was controlled, forty-five persons in the community suffered infection linked to these eight patients and to one other patient being held in juvenile hall.

I paged the hospital infection control nurse, informed her that we had a suspected meningococcal case, and gave her Jeremy's parents' names and telephone number. She passed on the information to the Los Angeles County Health Department. The key to stopping meningococcus from reaching epidemic proportions is to act faster than it can. During the week before he got sick, Jeremy had been heavily involved in a re-election campaign for a California State assemblywoman. He had been at campaign headquarters every day until the day he was admitted to the hospital, and on that particular day he had spent hours driving around Southern California with the candidate herself. Besides his family, the public health department had to track down over a hundred people so they could be given tablets of the antibiotic rifampin, to prevent meningococcal disease. (Antibiotics weren't necessary for us at the hospital because we had suspected the diagnosis from the beginning and had taken precautions.)

The next day was October 4. My intern Robert examined Jeremy and noted that he was still hypothermic and in shock. Robert added hydrocortisone by vein, in case the meningococcus had damaged Jeremy's adrenal glands. Then he went down to the x-ray department to meet me for rounds. While we were looking at the x-rays on the alternator, my beeper went off. It was the regional microbiology laboratory.

"Is this Dr. Nagami?" the voice at the other end asked.

"Yes."

"I have some positive blood cultures to report. The patient's name is Albright, first name Jeremy." She spoke slowly so I would get it right. "It looks like gram-negative diplococci in all six bottles."

"We suspected as much," I said. "And by the way, it's meningo-coccus, so be careful with it."

The next day, Jeremy started to have painful swelling in his ankles and in the small joints of his hands. This was a sign that he was beginning to recover from his meningococcal sepsis. His body was reacting to the large amount of antibody that he was manufac-turing against the invading bacteria. His pulse was now in the eight-ies, and his blood-clotting studies were back to normal. Robert and I were jubilant. "This is why you went to medical school!" I told him.

In the morning, Jeremy was able to move his ankles a little, al-though they were still painful. However, when he tried to stand, he found that he was extremely weak and dizzy. I arranged to have him evaluated by physical therapy and then went off to finish my morning clinic. It was Thursday and I was glad to leave at 12:30. It had been a hard five days.

That afternoon I taught a nutrition lesson to Ellen's fourth grade class. I divided everything that could be eaten into two columns with the headings, "Good for You, but Bad" and "Bad for You, but Good." Under the first column I listed foods like yogurt and broccoli, and under the second I put pizza, ice cream, and cheeseburgers. From these food groups, I explained to the class the balance that exists between good nutrition and human happiness. The children took notes while the teacher looked on in amazement.

On Friday, Jeremy went home. He had a deep ulcer on his right ankle where one of his purple lesions had caused gangrene (cell death) in the deeper tissues. This wound would require careful dressing by his mother. The rest of his spots were starting to fade.

His muscles and joints hurt badly. He needed ibuprofen and narcotic pain pills, but he was happy to leave the hospital for his own bed. Before he was discharged, the pharmacist gave Jeremy four rifampin pills to take, one twice a day for two days.

When I got home from work that Friday night, I found Ellen sick with a fever of over 103. Had I brought Jeremy's terrible disease home to my eight-year-old? Frantically, I looked over her body for a rash. Her skin was hot to the touch and she complained about being uncovered, but there were no telltale red, bleeding spots. I wrapped her up in blankets and went right back to the hospital. I told the pediatrician about Jeremy. He ordered blood and urine tests for Ellen, which were normal. I felt guilty for putting Ellen through the extra pain of a blood test, which wouldn't have been necessary if she'd been anyone else's kid. But I thought, "By saving lives I can keep families together, so it has to be worth it."

The next day was Saturday. Ellen woke up feeling better, though her temperature was 102. I was happy to be home to watch over her. I sorted through my collection of phonograph records. Then Ellen and I camped out on the living room couch, listening to old music, playing poker, and eating red licorice and potato chips.

It was several weeks before Jeremy could walk more than the short distance to the bathroom. His weakness was profound. Robert saw him in follow-up in his clinic and for a while it looked as if Jeremy might need a skin graft to cover the patch of gangrene on the side of his right ankle. But in the end, the area healed on its own. The waiting period passed and Jeremy's bone marrow was not injured by the chloramphenicol.

Since Jeremy's illness, the syndrome of meningococcal sepsis and meningitis caught the attention of the media when a number of fatal cases occurred among college students. Some of the survivors were not as fortunate as Jeremy had been and had to have limbs amputated as a result of gangrene. In fact, there is an increased risk of meningococcal disease in young persons living in group settings (barracks, prisons, and dormitories). The Advisory Committee on Immunization Practices is now recommending that administration of meningococcal vaccine be considered for college students living in dormitories. Vaccination is not routinely offered, however, and young people going off to college may have to specifically request it from their health care providers.

Meningococcal vaccine is made from the polysaccharide cell walls of dead meningococcal bacteria. It's safe and is 85 to 100 percent effective in adults in preventing invasive disease caused by *Neisseria meningitidis*, serogroups A and C. Unfortunately, another serogroup, type B, is responsible for many outbreaks in the United States and, for unknown reasons, the body does not respond very well to this polysaccharide in vaccines. So it's still very important for people to be aware of this terrible disease and to bring any patient with high fever and a rapidly spreading rash to the hospital as soon as possible. If Jeremy's mother had not acted so promptly, we would not have been able to save her son.

One evening about a year and a half after Jeremy's illness, I was working in the Urgent Care Clinic, when I saw his name among the stack of patient charts waiting to be seen. I picked up his chart and went to the room number written on the paperwork. I was delighted to see Jeremy sitting there, even if he was in a wheelchair. He held an x-ray and had a sheepish look on his face. While helping a friend move, he had dropped a dresser on his toe. The x-ray looked OK and nothing was fractured. I kneeled down to examine his foot; his big toe was bruised and swollen. My eyes moved to the outside of the ankle where I saw a deep, flame-shaped groove in the skin and underlying tissue. It was covered with a thin dark scar. I looked up at Jeremy and he looked gravely back at me. It was a permanent reminder of his narrow escape from a deadly infection.

conclusion

A few years ago I was in my neighborhood video store starting the
Friday night stroll down the rack of new releases when I heard
someone calling my name. It was Danielle, the woman who'd had
the worm in her brain. We exchanged greetings like any two people
meeting in a public place. No one could tell what we'd been through
together, or what a miracle Danielle's fluent speech was.

I see my patients around town all the time—and some of
them, like Jeremy, were so ill when I took care of them, that they
seem like spirits redeemed. But every redemption has its price, not
just for the one saved but for the one who brings them back.

Many years ago in medical school I made a decision not to
run away, to stay and witness terrible things, and because of this,
I've been able to help patients. But my experiences have made me
feel different from people outside medicine. I get close enough to
these diseases to know them intimately—their smells, their habits,
their textures—and, in a way, to become infected with them myself.
They get under my skin; they leave a telling mark. The things I've

seen divide me from others, making me, not more powerful, just different.

Medicine isn't about power, though a lot of people think that's what doctors feel. It's true we've come a long way since that day in 1924 when my Swiss Aunt Germaine arrived in Metz to begin her nurse's training. Then, a clean dressing and the surgeon's knife were the only defense against infection. But I don't think I feel more powerful today than she did. She knew she was at the beginning of a new age as she pioneered inhaled oxygen and attached the first patients to the electrocardiogram machine.

I didn't realize it, but I, too, was at the beginning of a new age when I started my internship in 1976. The first HIV-infected patients were already fanning out across the country, and our ability to promise a drug for every disease faded as we searched for ways to comfort the dying patients we couldn't help. A scant forty years into the age of antibiotics and we had already reached the upper limit of penicillin that could be injected into a patient to treat gonorrhea, and strains of the bacteria appeared that year that were completely insensitive to the drug. These gonococci were the harbingers of the highly antibiotic-resistant germs to come during my lifetime of practice. In another fifty years our treatment techniques in infectious disease—based on having a drug for every bug—may be of only historic interest.

But in the meantime, my colleagues and I will go on battling these diseases with the tools we have, always trying to keep a trick or two in reserve, like nimble chess players in match after match against ever-changing adversaries. If we're lucky we can outpace them, but it helps if we have a head start.

My hope in writing this book is not to create unnecessary fear, but rather to educate readers about the potential for danger lurking in everything from salads to the very air we breathe. To some degree, we all live with the illusion that it could never happen to us. We live in a modern world with a cure for almost everything. Even when we hear news stories about "flesh-eating strep" or deadly cases of meningococcus on a college campus we do so with a cool sense of detachment, assuming that there must have been something unusual about the victims. But the cases I've told you about, my patients, are mostly ordinary people just like you or me. Their experiences should serve as a warning that it can happen to any of us.

As I said at the beginning, I know things about the human body because I've looked at what lucky people never see. Through my story you've had an opportunity to observe from a safe distance some of the things I see and the way I see them. Hopefully, now if you haven't had chickenpox, you will get the vaccine, and if you live in cocci hot spots, you'll think twice before hiking in the hills on a windy day. The maneaters are out there, but you don't have to let them in.

glossary

Acquired Immunodeficiency Syndrome (AIDS): The condition caused by the human immunodeficiency virus (HIV). AIDS follows a long period of HIV infection, during which the immune system is damaged but few symptoms are apparent. AIDS may include infection, cancer, and weight loss and is eventually fatal if untreated.

Acute Respiratory Distress Syndrome (ARDS): A disorder of the lung tissue caused by infection, shock, burns, or other insults in which the capillaries become leaky and the air spaces fill with fluid.

Acyclovir: An antiviral drug that is active against the herpes virus causing herpes lesions of the mouth and genitals, herpes encephalitis, and chickenpox.

AIDS dementia complex: A disease of the brain caused by HIV. It includes slow thinking, decreased memory, and difficulties with speaking and walking.

Albendazole: A drug used to treat patients with parasitic infections.

Amebiasis: Infection with one-celled organisms (parasitic protozoa) called amebas. It is spread by contaminated food and drink and affects the colon and the liver.

Amphotericin B: An antibiotic used to treat serious fungal infections.

Amyl nitrate: A drug that dilates the blood vessels and is sometimes used recreationally.

Anemia, aplastic: A disease that results when the blood-forming cells in the bone marrow fail to grow and divide, causing a deficiency of blood cells (white blood cells, red blood cells, and platelets).

Anopheles: A genus of mosquitoes that transmits malaria.

Antibiotics: Drugs that inhibit or destroy microorganisms. They are ineffective against viruses.

Apharesis: A procedure in which a patient's blood is passed through a machine to exchange a specific component, such as plasma.

Apraxia: The inability to perform normally easy actions. Examples include the misuse of everyday objects due to misidentification and the inability to perform complex motions with the limbs.

ARDS: See Acute Respiratory Distress Syndrome.

Arthrospores: Spores produced by the dividing and breaking off of portions of fungi. The spores that cause coccidioidomycosis fall into this category.

Ascaris: An intestinal worm, which may grow to be over eight inches long.

Aspergillus: A genus of mold that can cause lung and brain infections in patients with weakened immune systems.

Attending physician: A senior physician who supervises physicians in training.

AZT: Zidovudine. The first drug developed to treat HIV. It is still useful in combination with other drugs.

Bacteria: Term for certain microorganisms that lack the ability to create food from light. They are larger than viruses and smaller than fungi and protozoa.

Bilirubin: A yellow pigment that results from the metabolism of the red blood cell protein, hemoglobin.

Black water fever: Kidney failure caused by malaria.

Candida albicans: An organism similar to yeast, C. albicans normally causes minor infections. However, it can cause serious infections in severely ill patients whose immune functions are weakened.

Centers for Disease Control (CDC): Now known as the Centers for Disease Control and Prevention, it is a federal government facility based in Atlanta, Georgia, that organizes monitoring and treatment programs for preventable diseases.

Cerebrospinal fluid: The clear, colorless fluid that surrounds the spinal cord and brain and fills the interior cavities of these structures.

Ceviche or seviche: Raw fish marinated in lime or lemon juice.

Chagas disease: A chronic parasitic disease of the heart and esophagus transmitted by biting bugs and caused by the protozoan parasite Trypanosoma cruzi.

Childbed fever: The old term for the infection of the reproductive organs and blood stream that commonly followed childbirth, particularly in contaminated settings. The usual cause was group A strep.

Chloramphenicol: An antibiotic that has been known to cause aplastic anemia in rare cases.

Chloroquine: An anti-malarial drug to which many strains of *Plasmodium falciparum* have now become resistant.

Cirrhosis of the liver: Irreversible liver damage with extensive scarring and distortion of normal structure, which interferes with liver function. Many agents, including toxins like alcohol and chronic viral infection, may cause cirrhosis.

Cisternal injection: An injection made at the base of the skull into the space where the brain stem meets the spinal cord.

CMV: See Cytomegalovirus.

Cobras: Venomous snakes of the genus *Naja*.

Cocci: See Coccidioidomycosis.

Cocci meningitis: A form of coccidioidomycosis that attacks the lining of the brain.

Coccidioidomycosis: The potentially fatal disease known as Valley Fever. Caused by inhalation of the spores of the fungus *Coccidioides immitis*, it can result in pneumonia and meningitis.

Coccidioidomycosis Serology Laboratory: A facility at the University of California at Davis that performs serological tests on the blood and cerebrospinal fluids of patients with coccidioidomycosis.

Commensal species: Two species that coexist with each other in such a way as to benefit one while the other is unaffected.

Creatinine: A component of urine that can accumulate in the blood if the kidneys are not working properly.

Cryptococcus: A fungus that causes infections in patients with weakened immune systems. It is contracted by inhaling fungal spores and affects the lungs and the brain.

CT scan: A computerized x-ray scan used to locate tissue damage.

Cyclops: A tiny organism that serves as the host for the larval form of the roundworm causing gnathostomiasis.

Cysticercosis: The disease caused by infection by the larval stage of the pork tapeworm, *Taenia solium.* It affects the brain, eyes, and muscles.

Cytomegalovirus (CMV): A virus in the herpes family that infects the retinas of AIDS patients, causing blindness.

Decadron: A drug in the steroid family that is used to decrease swelling in the brain.

Dengue fever: A viral disease transmitted by mosquitoes that causes pain in the head, joints, and muscles; fever; and sometimes bleeding.

Dialysis: The use of a machine that acts as an "artificial kidney" by filtering the blood or fluid introduced into the abdominal cavity.

Disseminated intravascular coagulation (DIC): Activation of blood-clotting factors and platelets inside the blood vessels throughout the body. It may be triggered by infection, burns, snake bite, or other factors and may result in uncontrolled bleeding due to depletion of these elements.

Dopamine: A drug given by vein to support blood pressure in patients in shock.

Doxycycline: An antibiotic in the tetracycline family active against many species of bacteria.

Drug allergy: An abnormal sensitivity to a medication, usually manifested by rash and sometimes fever.

Ebola: A viral hemorrhagic fever with a high mortality rate.

Echocardiogram: An image of the interior of the heart created by passing ultrasonic beams through the chest wall.

Echocardiogram, transesophageal: A procedure performed by placing an ultrasound probe inside the patient's esophagus to view the heart.

Electroencephalogram (EEG): The use of scalp electrodes to record the electrical activity of the brain.

Elephantiasis: A condition, often produced by roundworm parasites, in which obstruction to lymphatic drainage causes extreme swelling of the legs or the scrotum.

Embolus: A clot or foreign substance that is carried by the flow of blood from the central circulation and lodges in a smaller vessel causing obstruction to the flow of blood.

Encephalitis: An inflammatory condition of the brain tissue that may be produced by infectious agents.

Endocarditis, infectious: Inflammation of the heart lining or heart valves due to infection.

Endotracheal tube: A tube inserted in the windpipe so that a patient can breathe by artificial means.

Eosinophils: White blood cells that increase in number during allergic or parasitic illnesses. They are filled with granules that stain bright red with the dye eosin.

Espundia: A chronic destructive disease of the nose and mouth found chiefly in Brazil and caused by the protozoan parasite *Leishmania braziliensis.*

Exchange transfusion: A type of blood transfusion in which most of the patient's blood is exchanged for blood from various donors.

Falciparum malaria: The most dangerous form of malaria. It is caused by *Plasmodium falciparum* and is often resistant to treatment with common anti-malarial drugs.

Fasciitis, necrotizing: An invasive infection of the tissues and muscle that spreads along the connective tissues separating muscle groups (fascia) and leads to tissue death.

Filaria: Small parasitic roundworms transmitted by the bite of mosquitoes.

Flatworms: A group of worms that includes the flukes, tapeworms, and schistosomes as well as free-living forms, like the planaria.

Fluconazole: An antifungal drug.

Flukes: Several species of parasitic flatworms that inhabit the lungs, liver, intestines, and bladder.

Formalin: A solution of formaldehyde used for preserving tissue for study.

Fundi: Structures forming the back wall of the eye that are seen with an ophthalmoscope and include the retina and its blood vessels.

Fungi: Organisms that reproduce with spores and lack the ability to create food with light. They are larger than bacteria.

Gangrene: Tissue death caused by lack of blood flow. Certain bacterial infections produce gas gangrene in which gas is released into the dying tissues by the bacterial metabolism.

Germs: Bacteria that cause infectious diseases.

Glioma: A type of malignant brain tumor.

Gnathostoma spinigerum: The parasitic roundworm whose larva causes gnathostomiasis. The disease is transmitted by eating undercooked fish or snake. It affects the brain, the eye, the liver, and the tissues under the skin.

Gram-negative bacteria: Bacteria that turn pink when stained with Gram's stain. *Klebsiella* and the meningococcus are gram-negative bacteria.

Gram-positive bacteria: Bacteria that turn blue when stained with Gram's stain. Group A strep, the pneumococcus, and the staphylococcus are gram-positive.

Gram's stain: A method of staining devised by Dr. Christian Gram that is used to differentiate between various types of bacteria.

Granulation tissue: Small raised lumps of tissue that form in healing wounds.

Group A strep: See *Streptococcus pyogenes.*

Haemophilus aphrophilus: A gram-negative, rod-shaped bacterium that may cause infectious endocarditis.

Hemodialysis: See Dialysis.

Hemoglobin: The iron-containing protein that gives red blood cells their color and carries oxygen.

Hemorrhagic fevers: Infectious fevers that are complicated by spontaneous, uncontrolled bleeding.

Heroin: A narcotic drug related to morphine.

Herpes: A viral infection of the lips, skin, or genital areas that tends to recur. The same virus may cause encephalitis.

Hippocratic school: The proponents of the ideas of Hippocrates (460–377 B.C.), the physician who has been called the "Father of Medicine."

Human immunodeficiency virus (HIV): The virus that causes AIDS. It is transmitted by sexual contact, administration of contaminated blood products, childbirth, needle stick injury, and intravenous drug abuse.

Hydrocephalus, obstructive: An accumulation of cerebrospinal fluid within the brain caused by a blockage in its drainage pathways.

ID doctors: Doctors who specialize in infectious diseases.

Interferon alpha: A naturally occurring protein used to treat certain viral infections.

Itraconazole: An antifungal drug.

Kaposi's sarcoma: A reddish brown malignant tumor that usually begins in the skin, most commonly in patients with HIV. It has been linked to infection with a newly recognized virus, human herpes virus type 8.

Klebsiella: A bacterium normally present in the gut that can cause infections in the urine, lungs, and blood.

Kuru: A slow virus infection of the brain contracted by cannibalism.

Lateral cervical puncture: A procedure in which a needle is inserted into the neck below the ear to obtain cerebrospinal fluid or to administer drugs near the base of the brain.

Leishmania: Various protozoan parasites transmitted by biting flies that cause chronic infection of skin, mouth, nose, and internal organs.

Leukemia: A malignancy in which there is uncontrolled division of abnormal blood cells.

Lumbar puncture: Spinal tap. A procedure in which a needle is inserted into the small of the back to obtain cerebrospinal fluid for tests or to administer drugs.

M protein: A substance produced by group A strep that makes it resistant to destruction by white blood cells.

Mad cow disease: A slow virus disease of the brain affecting cows and people and transmitted by eating contaminated beef.

Magnetic Resonance Imaging (MRI): A method of imaging the body using a strong magnetic field.

Malaria: A mosquito-borne parasitic disease marked by recurring fever.

Malaria, falciparum: See Falciparum malaria.

Measles: A viral disease characterized by fever and a rash.

Meningitis: An inflammation of the lining of the brain or spinal cord.

Meningococcus: *Neisseria meningitis*, a gram-negative spherical bacterium that causes the sepsis syndrome and meningitis.

Mosquitoes: Insects that reproduce in still water. The female feeds on blood and transmits viral and parasitic diseases to animals and man.

MRI: See Magnetic Resonance Imaging.

Multiple sclerosis: A chronic condition of unknown cause in which nerve tissue in the brain and spinal cord is damaged by plaquelike scars.

Murmur: The sound produced when blood flows over abnormal areas of the heart.

Myoclonic jerk: A sharp, involuntary movement produced when brain function is momentarily impaired.

Neisseria meningitidis: See Meningococcus.

Nervous system, central: The brain, optic nerves, and spinal cord.

Neurocysticercosis: Brain, spinal cord, or eye infection by the larval form of the pork tapeworm, *Taenia solium*.

Non-nucleoside reverse transcriptase inhibitors: Drugs used for the treatment of HIV.

Obstetrics: The branch of medicine dealing with the management of pregnancy and childbirth.

Ommaya reservoir: A surgically implanted device that allows drugs to be injected into the fluid-filled cavity inside the brain via a rubber reservoir placed under the scalp.

Onchocerciasis: River blindness. Chronic infection by the roundworm *Onchocerca vulvulus*, which is transmitted by blackflies and is an important cause of blindness in Africa and Central and South America.

Oncospheres: The infectious larvae released from the eggs of the pork tapeworm.

Ophthalmoscope: A handheld instrument consisting of lighted lenses used to examine the interior of the eye.

Paragonimus: A flatworm in the fluke family that infects the lungs.

Parasite: An animal or vegetable organism that lives on or in another and draws its nourishment from its host.

Pediatrics: The branch of medicine dealing with the treatment of infants and children.

Penicillin: The first anti-microbial drug to be obtained from a mold.

Petechiae: Tiny spots of bleeding under the skin.

Phenobarbital: A drug in the barbiturate class used to treat and prevent seizures.

Planaria: Free-living flatworms that live in fresh water and in moist environments.

Plasma: The fluid portion of the blood that has not been allowed to clot.

Plasmodium: A genus of protozoan parasites that includes those causing human malaria.

Plasmodium falciparum: The parasite that causes falciparum malaria.

Platelets: The blood cell elements that aid in the clotting of blood.

Pneumocystis carinii: A one-celled parasite that causes pneumonia in malnourished infants, cancer patients, and patients with AIDS.

Pneumocystis carinii pneumonia (PCP): See Pneumocystis carinii.

Pneumonia: An inflammation of the lungs. Pneumococcal pneumonia, caused by *Streptococcus pneumoniae*, is the most common form of bacterial pneumonia.

Polymorphonuclear leukocytes (polys): White blood cells that attack and engulf microbial invaders in the blood stream.

Praziquantel: A drug active against parasitic worms.

Prosthetic: An artificial body part.

Protozoa: Single-cell organisms that are larger than bacteria and include both free-living forms and parasites. Parasitic protozoa include the agents of malaria, leishmaniasis, toxoplasmosis, and sleeping sickness (trypanosomiasis).

Pseudomonas aeruginosa: A gram-negative rod-shaped bacterium that infects open wounds, producing characteristic blue-green pus.

Purpuric fever: An infectious syndrome in which the patient develops fever and patches of bleeding under the skin, a hemorrhagic fever.

Pyrogenic exotoxins: Toxins produced by group A strep and by *Staphylococcus aureus* that cause fever, a scarlet fever rash, and the toxic shock syndrome that may follow infections with these microorganisms. They may function as superantigens.

Quinidine: A compound similar to quinine used to treat malaria and heart rhythm abnormalities.

Quinine: An anti-malarial drug obtained from the bark of the cinchona tree.

Rabies: A fatal viral infection of the brain (encephalitis) contracted from the bite or by other contact with the saliva of an infected animal.

Rheumatic fever: A disease caused by abnormal activation of the immune system following group A strep throat infection and characterized by fever, rash, arthritis, abnormal movements, and damage to the heart valves.

Rifampin: An antibiotic active against many microorganisms, including those causing tuberculosis.

River blindness: See Onchocerciasis.

Rocky Mountain Pus Club: A group of infectious disease doctors based in Idaho.

Rocky Mountain spotted fever: A dangerous hemorrhagic fever transmitted by tick bites and caused by a microorganism called a rickettsia.

Roth spot: A white spot surrounded by a red ring in the retina, visible through an ophthalmoscope, produced by an infected heart valve.

Roundworms: Primitive worms of variable size that may be free living or parasitic.

Rubella: German measles. A mild childhood disease, which, if acquired in the womb, may severely damage the heart and brain.

Scarlet fever: A disease produced by group A streptococcal toxins and characterized by fever and a bright red rash. Similar syndromes may occur in the staphylococcal toxic shock syndrome.

Schistosomiasis: A chronic disease, usually of the bladder or liver, caused by parasitic flatworms in the fluke family and transmitted by contact with larva released into fresh water by snails.

Sepsis: A life-threatening acute illness caused by blood stream invasion by microorganisms in which patients have various combinations of low blood pressure, destruction of blood-clotting elements, and failure of lungs, kidneys, and other organs.

Septic shock: Collapse of the normal blood pressure from blood stream invasion by microorganisms (sepsis).

Silvadene: An antibiotic cream applied to burned or severely damaged skin.

Slow virus infections: Infections of the brain produced by imperfect viruses or unusual infectious agents and preceded by incubation periods of many years.

Smallpox vaccine: A live-virus vaccine made from cowpox that confers protection against smallpox.

Sparganosis: An invasive infection by a larval tapeworm, often of the eye, contracted by applying a poultice made of raw frog flesh.

Spinal tap: See Lumbar puncture.

Spirometra: A species of larval tapeworm that is one of the causes of Sparganosis. See above.

Staphylococcus aureus: A gram-positive spherical bacterium that causes abscesses of the skin and that can invade the blood stream and infect any organ. It is also the cause of toxic shock syndrome associated with super-absorbent tampons.

Streptococcus pyogenes: Group A strep. A gram-positive spherical bacterium that produces many toxins that enable it to evade host defenses and to invade and damage tissues. It is the cause of "flesh-eating strep," strep throat, scarlet fever, and rheumatic fever.

Subacute Sclerosing Panencephalitis (SSPE): A slow virus infection of the brain caused by a defective form of the measles virus that occurs many years after measles.

Superantigens: Substances that are able to activate many immune functions at once, producing harmful effects in the patient, such as fever, shock, and organ failure. Pyrogenic exotoxins function as superantigens.

Syphilis: A disease transmitted sexually or in the womb and caused by a corkscrew-shaped bacterium that produces chronic infection of the brain, blood vessels, and other organs.

T helper cells: A type of white blood cell that is important in the body's defense against tuberculosis, herpes, and other infections, and which is destroyed by HIV.

Taenia solium: A tapeworm transmitted by inadequately cooked pork or by human hosts excreting its eggs in their stools. The adult worm causes intestinal infection. The larval worm may infect brain, eye, or muscle, a condition called cysticercosis.

Tapeworms: Parasitic flatworms whose adult forms live in the intestines and whose larval forms may infect the internal organs and brain.

Tegretol: A medication used to control seizures and other abnormal electrical discharges in the brain and nerves.

Toxic shock syndrome: An acute syndrome consisting of fever, low blood pressure, a red rash, and various combinations of confusion, watery diarrhea, kidney failure, liver failure, and a low platelet count. The largest outbreak was linked to super-absorbent tampons that became colonized with toxin-producing *Staphylococcus aureus*. Several toxins produced by these organisms play a role in the syndrome, including pyrogenic exotoxins similar to those implicated in group A strep syndromes.

Toxoplasmosis: A disease produced by a protozoan parasite and transmitted by undercooked meat and by cat feces. It affects the brain, eye, and heart.

Trichinosis: A disease of muscle caused by a parasitic roundworm and transmitted by eating undercooked pork or bear meat.

Tuberculosis: A bacterial infection of the lungs that may spread throughout the body. It is transmitted through the air from one person to another.

Typhoid: A bacterial infection caused by *Salmonella* and transmitted from one person to another or via food or water contaminated by an infected person who is excreting *Salmonella* in their stool. Patients have profound weakness and prolonged fever and may die without treatment.

Urechis caupo: A free-living burrowing marine worm that lives in tidal mudflats.

Valley Fever: A disease produced by inhaling spores of the fungus, *Coccidioides immitis,* affecting the lungs, skin, brain, and bones.

Valve, aortic: The heart valve between the left ventricle and the aorta that prevents the blood being pumped out of the heart from falling back into the left ventricle.

Valve, mitral: The heart valve between the right ventricle and the pulmonary artery that prevents the blood being pumped to the lungs from falling back into the right ventricle.

Valve, tricuspid: The heart valve between the right atrium and the right ventricle that prevents the blood being pumped to the lungs from being ejected backwards into the right atrium.

Varicella vaccine: A live-virus vaccine that confers protection against chickenpox.

Varicella virus (VZV): The virus in the herpes group that causes chickenpox and shingles.

Vegetations: In infectious endocarditis, collections of blood proteins and platelets adherent to heart valves that contain infecting microorganisms.

Ventilator: A machine used to deliver oxygenated air via a plastic tube into the lungs of a patient who is unable to breathe on his own.

Yellow fever: A viral infection transmitted by mosquitoes in which patients develop severe hepatitis.

Zidovudine: See AZT.

selected bibliography

books

Adams, Raymond D., and Maurice Victor. "Viral Infections of the Nervous System." In *Principles of Neurology*. 4th ed. New York: McGraw-Hill Information Services Co., 1989.

The American Heritage College Dictionary. 3d ed. Boston: Houghton Mifflin Co., 1993.

Barnes, Robert D. *Invertebrate Zoology*. Philadelphia: W. B. Saunders Co., 1968.

Binford, Chapman H., and Daniel H. Connor. *Pathology of Tropical and Extraordinary Diseases*. Vol. 2. Washington, D.C.: Armed Forces Institute of Pathology, 1976.

Buchsbaum, Ralph. *Animals Without Backbones*. 2d ed. Chicago: University of Chicago Press, 1974.

Einstein, Hans E. "Coccidioidomycosis of the Central Nervous System." In *Advances in Neurology*. Vol. 6. Edited by R. A. Thompson and J. R. Green. New York: Reven Press, 1974.

Garrett, Laurie. *The Coming Plague: Newly Emerging Diseases in a World Out of Balance.* New York: Penguin Books, 1994.

Houff, Sidney A., and John L. Seyer. "Slow Virus Diseases of the Central Nervous System." In *Disease-a-Month*, 22–31. Chicago: Year Book Medical Publishers, 1985.

Jong, Elaine C. *The Travel and Tropical Medicine Manual.* Philadelphia: W. B. Saunders Co., 1987.

Nagami, Pamela H., and Phyllis Guze. "Infectious Disease Emergencies." In *Current Emergency Diagnosis and Treatment.* 4th ed. Edited by Charles E. Saunders and Mary T. Ho, 605–646. Norwalk: Appleton and Lange, 1992.

Nouwen, Henri J. M. *The Wounded Healer.* Garden City: Image/ Doubleday, 1974.

Roueché, Berton. *The Orange Man: And Other Narratives of Medical Detection.* Boston: Little, Brown and Company, 1971.

Stedman's Medical Dictionary. 22d ed. Baltimore: The Williams and Wilkins Co., 1972.

Shilts, Randy. *And the Band Played On: Politics, People, and the AIDS Epidemic.* New York: Penguin Books, 1988.

Thurman, Judith. *Isak Dinesen: The Life of a Storyteller.* New York: St. Martin's Press, 1982.

U.S. Census Bureau. *Statistical Abstract of the United States: 1999.* 119th ed. Washington, D.C.: U.S. Department of Commerce, 1999.

Vieusseux, Gaspard. "The Disease Which Raged in Geneva During the Spring of 1805." In *Classic Descriptions of Disease.* 3d ed. Edited by Ralph H. Major, 188–89. Springfield: Charles C. Thomas, 1978.

Warren, Kenneth S., and Adel Al Mahmoud. *Tropical and Geographical Medicine.* 2d ed. New York: McGraw-Hill Information Services Co., 1984.

Articles

Anlar, Banu, Kalbiye Yalaz, Ferhunde Öktem, and Gülsen Köse. "Long-Term Follow-up of Patients with Subacute Sclerosing Panencephalitis Treated with Intraventricular Alpha-Interferon." *Neurology* 48 (February 1997): 526–28.

Barré-Sinoussi, F., J. C. Chermann, F. Rey, M. T. Nugeyre, S. Chamaret, J. Gruest, C. Dauguet, C. Axler-Blin, F. Vézinet-Brun, C. Rouzioux, W. Rosenbaum, and L. Montagnier. "Isolation of a T-Lymphotropic Retrovirus from a Patient at Risk for Acquired Immune Deficiency Syndrome (AIDS)." *Science* 220 (May 20, 1983): 868–71.

Berbari, Elie F., Franklin R. Cockerill, and James A. Steckelberg. "Infective Endocarditis Due to Unusual or Fastidious Microorganisms." *Mayo Clinic Proceedings* 72 (June 1997): 532–42.

Bieger, Cyril, Nelson S. Brewer, and John A. Washington II. "Hemophilus Aphrophilus: A Microbiologic and Clinical Review and Report of 42 Cases." *Medicine* (Baltimore) 57, no. 4 (1978): 345–55.

Bouza, Emilio, Jerrold S. Dreyer, William L. Hewitt, and Richard D. Meyer. "Coccidioidal Meningitis." *Medicine* (Baltimore) 60, no. 3 (1981): 139–72.

Burr, Ty. "The Death of Jim Henson." *Entertainment Weekly,* no. 379 (May 16, 1997): 132.

Case Records of the Massachusetts General Hospital (Case 25-1986). *New England Journal of Medicine* 314, no. 26 (June 26, 1986): 1689–1700.

CDC. "Advisory Committee on Immunization Practices (ACIP) Modifies Recommendations for Meningitis Vaccination." Division of Media Relations (404) 639-3286, Press Release October 21, 1999.

————. "Coccidioidomycosis Following the Northridge Earthquake—
California, 1994." *Morbidity and Mortality Weekly Report* 43, no. 10
(March 18, 1994): 194–95.

————. "Imported Dengue—United States, 1997 and 1998." *Morbidity
and Mortality Weekly Report* 49, no. 12 (March 31, 2000): 248–53.

————. "Outbreak of West Nile–like Viral Encephalitis—New York,
1999." *Morbidity and Mortality Weekly Report* 49, no. 12 (March 31,
2000): 248–53.

————. "Prevention of Varicella: Update Recommendations of the
Advisory Committee on Immunization Practices (ACIP)." *Morbidity
and Mortality Weekly Report* 48, no. RR-6 (May 28, 1999): 1–5.

————. "Treatment with Quinidine Gluconate of Persons with Severe
Plasmodium Falciparum Infection: Discontinuation of Parenteral
Quinine from CDC Drug Service." *Morbidity and Mortality Weekly
Report* 40, no. RR-4 (June 1992): 21–23.

————. "Varicella-Related Deaths among Adults—United States, 1997."
Morbidity and Mortality Weekly Report 46, no. 19 (May 16, 1997):
409–12.

Charles, David, and Bryan Larsen. "Streptococcal Puerperal Sepsis and
Obstetric Infections: A Historical Perspective." *Reviews of
Infectious Diseases* 8, no. 3 (May–June 1986): 411–21.

Como, Jackson A., and William E. Dismukes. "Oral Azole Drugs as
Systemic Antifungal Therapy." *New England Journal of Medicine*
330, no. 4 (January 27, 1994): 263–72.

Cruz, Marcelo, Juan Cruz, and John Horton. "Albendazole versus
Praziquantel in the Treatment of Cerebral Cysticercosis: Clinical
Evaluation." *Transactions of the Royal Society of Tropical Medicine
and Hygiene* 85 (1991): 244–47.

DeGhetaldi, Lawrence C., Robert M. Norman, and Arthur W.
    Douville. "Cerebral Cysticercosis Treated Biphasically with
    Dexamethasone and Praziquantel." *Annals of Internal Medicine*
    1983, no. 2 (August 1983): 179–82.

Demers, B., A. E. Simor, H. Vellend, P. M. Schlievert, S. Byrne,
    F. Jamieson, S. Walmsley, and D. E. Low. "Severe Invasive Group
    A Streptococcal Infections in Ontario, Canada: 1987–1991." *Clinical
    Infectious Diseases* 16 (June 1993): 792–802.

Dewsnup, Daniel H., John N. Galgiani, J. Richard Graybill, Manuel
    Diaz, Adrian Rendon, Gretchen A. Cloud, and David A. Stevens.
    "Is It Ever Safe to Stop Azole Therapy for Coccidioides Immitis
    Meningitis?" *Annals of Internal Medicine* 124, no. 3 (February 1,
    1996): 305–10.

DiPersio, Joseph R., Thomas M. File Jr., Dennis L. Stevens, William G.
    Gardner, George Petropoulos, and Kawaljit Dinsa. "Spread of
    Serious Disease-Producing M3 Clones of Group A Streptococcus
    Among Family Members and Health Care Workers." *Clinical
    Infectious Diseases* 22 (March 1996): 490–95.

Drutz, David J., and Antonino Catanzaro. "Coccidioidomycosis."
    American Review of Respiratory Diseases 117 (1978): 559–85, 727–71.

Drutz, David J., and Milton Huppert. "Coccidioidomycosis: Factors
    Affecting the Host-Parasite Interaction." *Journal of Infectious
    Diseases* 147, no. 3 (March 1983): 372–90.

Dunn, Ruth Ann. "Subacute Sclerosing Panencephalitis." *Pediatric
    Infectious Disease Journal* 10, no. 1 (January 1991): 68–71.

Dyken, Paul R. "Subacute Sclerosing Panencephalitis." *Neurology Clinics*
    3, no. 1 (February 1985): 179–96.

Dyken, P., M. Philippart, and P. Maertens. "The Chronic Progressive Encephalitides of Childhood." *Neurological Infections and Epidemiology* 2, no. 2 (1997): 145–58.

Einstein, Hans E. "Coccidioidomycosis: New Aspects of Epidemiology and Therapy." *Clinical Infectious Diseases* 16 (March 1993): 349–54.

Fauci, Anthony S. "The AIDS Epidemic: Considerations for the 21st Century." *New England Journal of Medicine* 341, no. 14 (September 30, 1999): 1046–50.

Feigin, Ralph D., Carol J. Baker, Lureen A. Herwaldt, Richard M. Lampe, Edward O. Mason, and Stephen E. Whitney. "Epidemic Meningococcal Disease in an Elementary-School Classroom." *New England Journal of Medicine* 307, no. 20 (November 11, 1982): 1255–57.

Formenty, Pierre, Christophe Boesch, Monique Wyers, Claudia Steiner, Franca Donati, Frédéric Dind, Francine Walker, and Bernard Le Geunno. "Ebola Virus Outbreak among Wild Chimpanzees Living in a Rain Forest of Côte d'Ivoire." *Journal of Infectious Diseases* 179, Supplement 1 (1999): S120– 126.

Formenty, Pierre, Christopher Hatz, Bernard Le Guenno, Agnés Stoll, Philipp Rogenmoser, and Adreas Widmer. "Human Infection Due to Ebola Virus, Subtype Côte d'Ivoire: Clinical and Biologic Presentation." *Journal of Infectious Diseases* 179, Supplement 1 (1999): S48–S53.

Forni, Arthur L., Edward L. Kaplan, Patrick M. Schlievert, and Richard B. Roberts. "Clinical and Microbiological Characteristics of Severe Group A Streptococcus Infections and Streptococcal Toxic Shock Syndrome." *Clinical Infectious Diseases* 21 (August 1995): 333–40.

Fradin, Mark S. "Mosquitoes and Mosquito Repellants: A Clinician's Guide." *Annals of Internal Medicine* 128, no. 11 (June 1, 1998): 931–40.

Galgiani, John N., Antonino Catanzaro, Gretchen A. Cloud, Jean
    Higgs, Barry A. Friedman, Robert A. Larsen, John R. Graybill,
    and the NIAID Mycosis Study Group. "Fluconazole Therapy in
    the Treatment of Coccidioidal Meningitis." *Annals of Internal
    Medicine* 119, no. 1 (July 1, 1993): 28–35.

Gallo, Robert C., Syed Z. Salahuddin, Mikulas Popovic, Gene M.
    Shearer, Mark Kaplan, Barton F. Haynes, Thomas J. Palker, Robert
    Redfield, James Oleske, Bijan Safai, Gilbert White, Paul Foster,
    and Phillip D. Markham. "Frequent Detection and Isolation of
    Cytopathic Retroviruses (HTLV-III) from Patients with AIDS
    and at Risk for AIDS." *Science* 224 (May 4, 1984): 500–502.

Garg, R. K., B. Karak, and A. M. Sharma. "Subacute Sclerosing
    Panencephalitis." *Indian Pediatrics* 35, (April 1998): 337–45.

Gottlieb, Michael S., Robert Shroff, Howard M. Schanker, Joel D.
    Weisman, Peng Thim Fan, Robert A. Wolf, and Andrew Saxon.
    "Pneumocystis Carinii Pneumonia and Mucosal Candidiasis in
    Previously Healthy Homosexual Men." *New England Journal of
    Medicine* 305, no. 24 (December 10, 1981): 1425–38.

Hook, Edward W., III. "Gonococcal Infections." *Annals of Internal
    Medicine* 102, no. 2 (February 1985): 225–43.

Huttenlocher, P. R., D. L. Picchietti, R. P. Roos, N. R. Cashman,
    B. Horowitz, and M. S. Horowitz. "Intrathecal Interferon in
    Subacute Sclerosing Panencephalitis." *Annals of Neurology* 19
    (1986): 303–305.

Jackson, Mary Anne, V. Fred Burry, and Lloyd C. Olson. "Multisystem
    Group A Beta-Hemolytic Streptococcal Disease in Children."
    Reviews of Infectious Diseases 13 (September–October 1991):
    783–788.

Kraivichian, Phisai, Medhi Kulkumthorn, Paisal Yingyourd, Penkae
    Akarabovorn, and Chaun-Chuin Paireepai. "Albendazole for the
    Treatment of Human Gnathostomiasis." *Transactions of the Royal
    Society for Tropical Medicine and Hygiene* 86, no. 4 (July 8, 1992):
    418–21.

Loo, Lawrence, and Abraham Braude. "Cerebral Cysticercosis in San
    Diego: A Report of 23 Cases and a Review of the Literature."
    Medicine (Baltimore) 61, no. 6 (1982): 341–59.

McDonald, Malcolm I., G. Ralph Corey, Harry A. Gallis, and David T.
    Durack. "Single and Multiple Pyogenic Liver Abscesses, Natural
    History, Diagnosis and Treatment, with Emphasis on
    Percutaneous Drainage." *Medicine* (Baltimore) 63, no. 5 (1984):
    291–302.

Maimone, D., L. M. E. Grimaldi, G. Incorpora, R. Biondi, V. Sofia,
    G. Russo Mancuso, L. Siciliano, M. Ruscica, and L. Pavone.
    "Intrathecal Interferon in Subacute Sclerosing Panencephalitis."
    Acta Neurologica Scandinavia 78 (1988): 161–66.

Medical Staff Conference, University of California, San Francisco.
    "Meningococcus." *Western Journal of Medicine* 127, no. 4 (October
    1977): 314–24.

Miller, Kirk D., Alan E. Greenberg, and Carlos C. Campbell. "Treat-
    ment of Severe Malaria in the United States with a Continuous
    Infusion of Quinidine Gluconate and Exchange Transfusion." *New
    England Journal of Medicine* 321 (July 13, 1989): 65–70.

Nopparatana, C., W. Chaicumpa, P. Tapchaisri, P. Setasuban, and
    Y. Ruangkunaporn. "Towards a Suitable Antigen for Diagnosis of
    Gnathostoma Spinigera Infection." *Indian Journal of Parasitology*
    22, no. 8 (December 1992): 1151–56.

Pappagianis, Demosthenes, and Hans Einstein. "Tempest from
    Tehachapi Takes Toll or Coccidioides Conveyed Aloft and Afar."
    Western Journal of Medicine 129 (December 1978): 527–30.

Ratcheson, Robert A., and Ayub K. Ommaya. "Experience with the
    Subcutaneous Cerebrospinal Fluid Reservoir: A Preliminary
    Report of 60 Cases." *New England Journal of Medicine* 270, no. 19
    (November 7, 1968): 1025–31.

Richardson, K., K. Cooper, M. S. Marriott, M. H. Tarbit., P. F. Troke,
    and P. J. Whittle. "Discovery of Fluconazole, A Novel Antifungal
    Agent." *Reviews of Infectious Diseases* 12, Supplement 3
    (March–April 1990): 5267–71.

Rothenberg, Marc E. "Eosinophilia." *New England Journal of Medicine*
    338, no. 22 (May 28, 1998): 1592–600.

Rusnak, J. M., and D. R. Lucey. "Clinical Gnathostomiasis: Case Report
    and Review of the English-language Literature." *Clinical Infectious
    Diseases* 16, no. 1 (January 1993): 33–50.

Schantz, Peter M., Anne C. Moore, José L. Muñoz, Barry J. Hartman,
    John A. Schaeffer, Alan M. Aron, Deborah Persaud, Elsa Sarti,
    Marianna Wilson, and Ana Flisser. "Neurocysticercosis in an
    Orthodox Jewish Community in New York City." *New England
    Journal of Medicine* 327, no. 10 (September 3, 1992): 692–702.

Sherman, Ronald A., Joseph Silva, and Regina Gandour-Edwards.
    "Fatal Varicella in an Adult: Case Report and Review of the
    Gastrointestinal Complications of Chickenpox." *Reviews of
    Infectious Diseases* 13 (May–June 1991): 424–27.

Singer, Carlos, Anthony E. Lang, and Oksana Suchowersky. "Adult-Onset
    Subacute Sclerosing Panencephalitis: Case Reports and Review of
    the Literature." *Movement Disorders* 12, no. 3 (May 1997): 342–53.

Sotelo, Julio, Francisco Escobedo, Jesus Rodriguez-Carbajal, Bertha
    Torres, Franciso Rubio. "Therapy of Parenchymal Brain
    Cysticercosis with Praziquantel." *New England Journal of Medicine*
    310, no. 16 (April 19, 1984): 1001–1007.

Spicer, Thomas E., and Jerold M. Rau. "Purpura Fulminans." *American
    Journal of Medicine* 61 (October 1996): 566–71.

Stevens, Dennis L. "Invasive Group A Streptococcus Infections."
    Clinical Infectious Diseases 14 (January 1992): 2–11.

Stevens, Dennis L., Martha H. Tanner, Jay Winship, Raymond Swarts,
    Kristen M. Ries, Patrick M. Schlievert, and Edward Kaplan.
    "Severe Group A Streptococcal Infections Associated with a Toxic
    Shock–like Syndrome and Scarlet Fever Toxin A." *New England
    Journal of Medicine* 321, no. 1 (July 6, 1989): 1–12.

Suntharasamai, P., M. Riganti, S. Chittamas, and V. Desakorn.
    "Albendazole Stimulates Outward Migration of *Gnathostoma
    Spinigerum* to the Dermis in Man." *Southeast Asian Journal of
    Tropical Public Health* 23, no. 4 (December 1992): 716–22.

Tan, E., I. J. Namer, A. Ciger, T. Zileli, and T. Kucukali. "The Prognosis
    of Subacute Sclerosing Panencephalitis in Adults: Report of 8
    Cases and Review of the Literature." *Clinical Neurology and
    Neurosurgery* 93, no. 3 (1991): 205–209.

Tappero, Jordan W., R. Reporter, Jay D. Wenger, Bridget A. Ward,
    Michael W. Reeves, Timms Missbach, Brian D. Plikaytis, Laurene
    Mascula, and Anne Schuchat. "Meningococcal Disease in Los
    Angeles County, California, among Men in the County Jails." *New
    England Journal of Medicine* 335, no. 12 (September 19, 1996):
    833–40.

Temesgen, Zelalem, and Alan J. Wright. "Antiretrovirals." *Mayo Clinic*

Proceedings 74 (December 1999): 1284–301.

Terrell, Christine L. "Antifungal Agents, Part II: The Azoles." *Mayo Clinic Proceedings* 74 (January 1999): 78–100.

Trousseau, A. "Scarlatina." Reprinted from *Lectures on Clinical Medicine* by A. Trousseau, trans. J. R. Cormack and P. V. Bazire. 2 vols., Philadelphia: Lindsay and Blakiston, 1873, reprinted in *Reviews of Infectious Diseases* 1, no. 6 (November–December 1979): 1016–26.

Valenzuela, Terence D., Thomas M. Hooten, Edward L. Kaplan, and Patrick Schlievert. "Transmission of 'Toxic Strep' Syndrome from an Infected Child to a Firefighter During CPR." *Annals of Emergency Medicine* 20, no. 1 (January 1991): 90–92.

Vargas-Ocampo, Francisco, Eliseo Alarcón-Rivera, and Francisco J. Alvarado-Alemán. "Human Gnathostomiasis in Mexico." *International Journal of Dermatology* 37, no. 6 (June 1998): 441–44.

Vieira, Jeffrey, Elliot Frank, Thomas J. Spira, and Sheldon H. Landesman. "Acquired Immune Deficiency Syndrome in Haitians." *New England Journal of Medicine* 308, no. 3 (January 20, 1983): 125–129.

Vincent, Tom, John N. Galgiani, Milton Huppert, and David Salkin. "The Natural History of Coccidioidal Meningitis: VA-Armed Forces Cooperative Studies, 1955–1958." *Clinical Infectious Diseases* 16, no. 2 (February 1993): 243–54.

Virk, Abinash, and James M. Steckelberg. "Clinical Aspects of Anti-microbial Resistance." *Mayo Clinic Proceedings* 75 (February 2000): 200–14.

Wheeler, Arthur P., and Gordon R. Bernard. "Treating Patients with Severe Sepsis." *New England Journal of Medicine* 340, no. 3 (January 21, 1999): 207–14.

White, C. Jo. "Varicella-Zoster Virus Vaccine." *Clinical Infectious*

Diseases 24 (May 1997): 753–63.

Wilson, Marianna, Ralph T. Bryan, Janet A. Fried, Doris A. Ware, Peter M. Shantz, Joy B. Pilcher, and Victor C. W. Tsang. "Clinical Evaluation of the Cysticercosis Enzyme-linked Immuno-electrotransfer Blot in Patients with Neurocysticercosis." *Journal of Infectious Diseases* 164 (November–December 1991): 1007–1009.

Witorsch, Philip, and Philip Gorden. "Hemophilus Aphrophilus Endocarditis." *Annals of Internal Medicine* 60, no. 6 (June 1964): 957–61.

Yoshikawa, Thomas, Kouichi Tanaka, and Lucien B. Guze. "Infection and Disseminated Intravascular Coagulation." *Medicine* (Baltimore) 50, no. 4 (1971): 237–58.

index

about the author

Pamela Nagami received her M.D. degree from Yale University in 1976. She is a clinical associate professor of medicine at the UCLA School of Medicine and staff physician in internal medicine and infectious diseases with the Southern California Permanente Medical Group. She practices at the Kaiser Foundation Hospital in Woodland Hills, California.

Dr. Nagami is the author of book chapters, articles, and abstracts within her specialty. *The Woman with a Worm in Her Head* is her first book written for the general public. She lives with her husband, Glenn Nagami, M.D., and their two children in Encino, California.